Atlas of Pediatric Cutaneous Biodiversity

Nanette B. Silverberg

Atlas of Pediatric Cutaneous Biodiversity

Comparative Dermatologic Atlas
of Pediatric Skin of All Colors

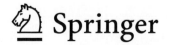 Springer

Nanette B. Silverberg, MD
Clinical Professor of Dermatology
Columbia University College of Physicians and Surgeons
Director, Pediatric and Adolescent Dermatology
St. Luke's-Roosevelt Hospital and Beth Israel Medical Centers
Department of Dermatology
1090 Amsterdam Avenue, Suite 11D
New York, NY 10025, USA

ISBN 978-1-4614-3563-1   e-ISBN 978-1-4614-3564-8
DOI 10.1007/978-1-4614-3564-8
Springer New York Heidelberg Dordrecht London

Library of Congress Control Number: 2012937072

Printed on acid-free paper

Springer is part of Springer Science+Business Media (www.springer.com)

This book is dedicated to all the people who have supported me through my career:

To my parents, who have always fostered creativity and intellectual growth

To my son, who taught me more about developmental pediatrics than I could have ever learned from a book, and in the happiest of ways

And to Dr. Teresita A. Laude, my first teacher on this subject, who generously lent her slides to this work

Preface

The intent of this atlas is to provide a foundation for comparative understanding of pediatric skin diseases between all the races and ethnicities. In this way, we can be better equipped to deal with a future of cutaneous biodiversity in which the majority of our patients will be of color, and where Caucasians will soon be a minority of the population, as they are now in most countries worldwide. Gaps in published literature on racial and ethnic variations do exist, and I try to identify these so that investigators with interest in Pediatric Dermatology can gear future research to filling in these gaps.

New York, NY, USA   Nanette B. Silverberg

Acknowledgments

I would like to thank the following individuals who were kind enough to offer their expert thoughts and ideas regarding specific topics:

Vincent De Leo, MD
Ilona Frieden, MD
Ashfaq Marghoob, MD
Richard Mizuguchi, MD
Lauren Pachman, MD
Amy Paller, MD
Robert Sidbury, MD, MPH
Jonathan I. Silverberg, MD, PhD, MPH

Contents

Fitzpatrick Phototyping Scale (Table 1.1)

Table 1.1 reviews the standard Fitzpatrick skin types as they may apply to children by race and ethnicity. The table also includes potential skin issues that are commonly noted in my clinical practice, based on these skin tones, race, and ethnicity.

Caucasian-Normal Skin Tone (Newborn) (Figs. 1.1 and 1.2)

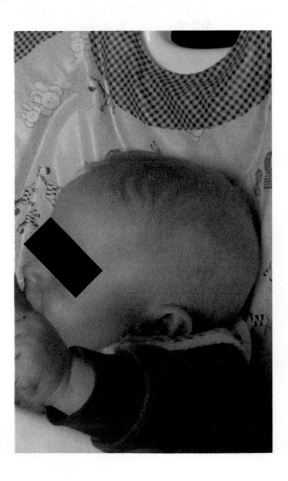

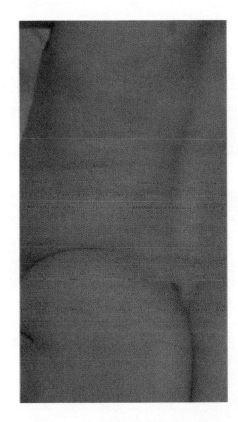

The normal skin of a newborn Caucasian child (Fig. 1.1) is lightly pigmented and can demonstrate light colored vellus hairs, prominent vasculature (Fig. 1.3), and easy formation of erythema with trauma. Furthermore, cutis marmorata can be prominent on the dependent portions of the body. Early changes that can be noted include milia, sebaceous hyperplasia, and infantile acne (Chap. 2). In early childhood, the skin loses much of the vascular reactivity patterns of infancy.

N.B. Silverberg, *Atlas of Pediatric Cutaneous Biodiversity: Comparative Dermatologic Atlas of Pediatric Skin of All Colors*, DOI 10.1007/978-1-4614-3564-8_1, © Springer Science+Business Media, LLC 2012

Table 1.1 Typical reaction patterns noted by race and ethnicity

Race/ethnicity	Fitzpatrick types	Skin reactions
Asian/East Asian	II–IV	Risk of sun damage, dyspigmentation, facial sensitivity, and keloids

Black/African American/Afro-Carribean	IV–VI	Risk of dyspigmentation, especially
		    Hyperpigmentation
		    Obfuscation of diagnosis due to pigmentary alterations
		    Xerosis
		    Keloids
		    Traction/styling hair damage

Caucasian	I, II (rarely III)	Risk of phototoxic reactions, damage, and vascular reactivity in response to trauma and ultraviolet light exposure
South east Asian/Indian	III–V	Risk of pigmentary disturbance, especially hypopigmentation Xerosis
Hispanic/Latino	II–V	Risk of dyspigmentation, both hyperpigmentation and hypopigmentation, obfuscation of diagnosis due to pigmentary alterations, xerosis, traction-related hair damage, keloids, and photodamage
Native American	II–IV	Risk of dyspigmentation, both hyperpigmentation and hypopigmentation, xerosis, obfuscation of diagnosis due to pigmentary alterations and photodamage
Middle Eastern	III–VI	Risk of dyspigmentation, both hyperpigmentation and hypopigmentation, xerosis, obfuscation of diagnosis due to pigmentary alterations and photodamage

Modified from Silverberg NB. Pediatric dermatology in children of color. Access Dermatol. 2010

Caucasian-Postdates Peeling (Figs. 1.3 and 1.4)

Postdates peeling is common in children who are 40 or more weeks gestational age and can range from a branny to thick coating of shiny hyperkeratosis, resembling the thicker encasements of collodion membranes. Accompanying hyperlinearity of the palms and soles can be noted (Fig. 1.3).

Dermoscopy demonstrates desquamation of the tiny stratum corneum keratinocytes around the edges (Fig. 1.4). Erythema noted in the background is a normal form of cutis marmorata of infancy, most obvious in Caucasian infants.

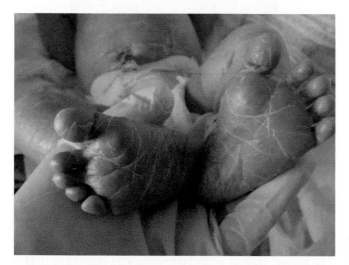

Hispanic/Latino-Normal Skin Tone (Newborn) (Figs. 1.5 and 1.6)

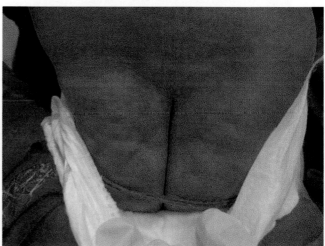

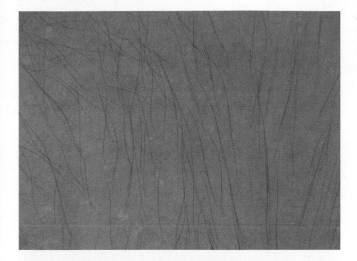

Fine lanugo and/or vellus hairs and mild desquamation of keratinocytes (Fig. 1.5), especially around follicular orifices, typifies newborn Hispanic/Latino skin. Lanugo hairs (Fig. 1.6) are noted in premature infants as they disappear towards the end of the third trimester, replaced by vellus hairs. Lanugo hairs and infantile vellus hairs are generally dark brown in this group of children as noted on the lower back in the Hispanic infant pictured in Figs. 1.5 and 1.6 (dermoscopic photo of the lower back seen in Fig. 1.5). Vellus hairs will usually disappear in the first year of life. However, some hirsute Hispanic/Latino children may have notable persistence of fine dark body hair over the trunk, back, and extremities through childhood. Congenital hairy pinna can be noted in infants of mothers with maternal gestational diabetes mellitus, but is also more common in individuals from the South Pacific, India, and Sri Lanka, as well as in some populations of Europe, Africa, and Australia [2].

Black/African American Normal Skin Tone (Newborn) (Fig. 1.7)

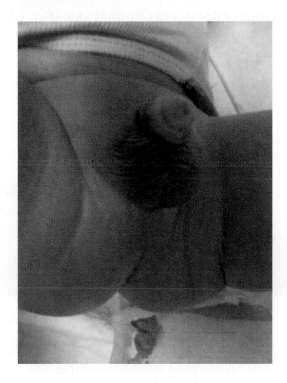

In newborns of Black, African American or Afro-Caribbean descent hyperpigmentation can be noted over the ears, lips, fingertips, genitalia (Fig. 1.7) (especially in the midline), nipples, umbilicus, axillae, and anal orifice. Only axillary hyperpigmentation disappears by the end of the first year [3]. Pigmentation of the body develops to its full depth of color through early childhood in Black children. During the first year of development, extreme lability in the form of hypopigmentation from insults is

Table 1.2 Ultrastructural differences in melanocyte distribution and melanosome packaging by race and ethnicity

Race	Pigmentary differences
Black (in the United States: African American or Afro-Caribbean)	Large (stage IV), dispersed melanosomes
	Eumelanin
	Closely packed doublet or singlet melanosomes, rare aggregates [4]. Larger melanophages (May account in part for greater incidence of melasma and erythema Dyschromicum Perstans)
	UV filtration in the malpighian layer
Asian	Mixed small and large melanosomes
	Aggregates in non-sun-exposed skin; nonaggregated in sun-exposed skin
Caucasian	Small, aggregated melanosomes
	Pheomelanin
	Few small melanophages
	UV filtration in the stratum corneum

common. Later on, hyperpigmentation prevails as a side effect of trauma (Table 1.2).

Caucasian Adolescents Normal Skin (Fig. 1.8)

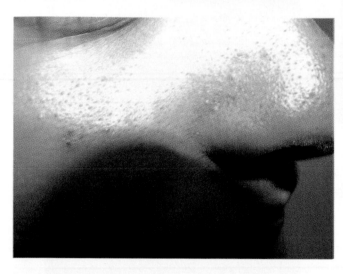

In adolescence, sebum production and hormonal influences can cause sheen and follicular "enlargement" of the sebaceous follicles or "pores" in the vernacular, which is actually a blockage causing increased prominence (Fig. 1.8).

Hispanic-Adolescents Normal Skin (Fig. 1.9)

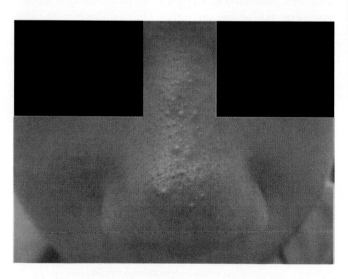

In this Hispanic/Latino adolescent, a mixture of occluded pores and retention of facial hairs, i.e., trichostasis spinulosa mark early adolescence (Fig. 1.9). Hyperkeratosis of the follicular orifices is prominent and topical retinoid therapy or salicyclic acid may be helpful in reversing these changes.

African American Adolescents Normal Skin (Figs. 1.10 and 1.11)

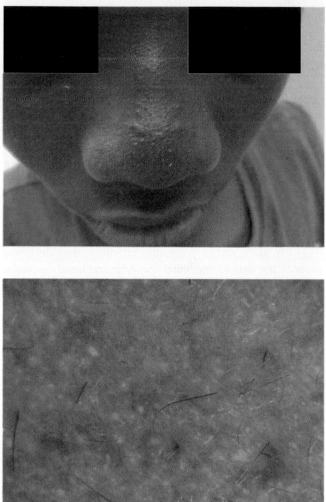

Follicular prominence of adolescence (Fig. 1.10) in this teenager results in a light halo near each sebaceous hair follicle of the face. This child has allergies and has developed pseudoacne of the nasal crease as well. Figure 1.11 demonstrates dermoscopy of an older adolescent with enlarged sebaceous glands and blocked follicular orifices. Some studies have suggested that sebum, the oil produced by sebaceous glands, has greater lipid content in Black individuals and that the sebaceous glands are larger in Black than Caucasians [4–6]. This may possibly allow for greater bacterial and yeast overgrowth.

Dorsal/Ventral Demarcation (Fig. 1.12)

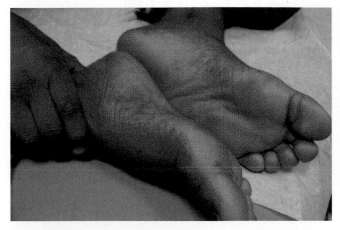

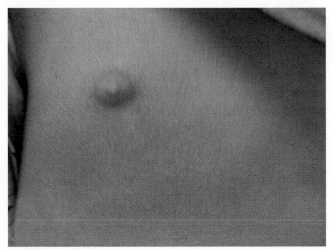

Light pigmentation of the plantar skin is notable in all racial and ethnic groupings; however, the difference in pigment between the dorsal and ventral surfaces is most marked in Black and Indian individuals (Fig. 1.12).

Skin Demarcation (Figs. 1.13–1.15)

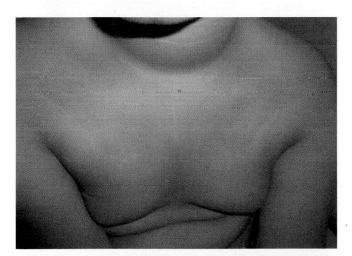

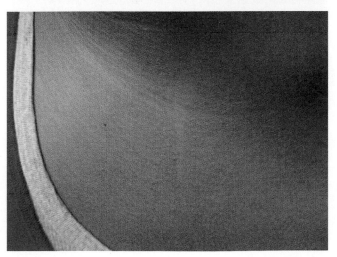

Langer's lines are skin cleavage lines, as would be noted in surgical procedures. Langer's lines show a laddering pattern of melanocytes as opposed to the standard honeycomb that is noted in most patients of color on the back. This may contribute to enhanced lesion healing and improved pigmentation when Langer's lines are observed [7].

Marginal skin pigmentation can be termed pigmentary demarcation lines of the B type as well. Seventy nine percent of adult Black women have pigmentary demarcation lines, types A (Fig. 1.13) or B accounting for 50%, with induction in pregnancy of type B lines in 14%. Seventy-five percent of Black males have pigmentary demarcation lines with type C being the most common. Only 15% of Caucasians have notable pigmentary demarcation lines [8] (Table 1.3).

Pigmentation lines are not noted in Caucasian neonates, but 46% of Black female infants will have pigmentary demarcation lines [8] including A (19%); B (27%); C (15%) (Fig. 1.14); D (1%); and E (1%) (Fig. 1.15), and 16% of Black male infants including A (8%) and B (8%). In childhood, the numbers increase for Black children, including 63% of Black females (A 36%, B 0%, C 45%, D 0%, E 1%) and 87% of Black males (A 50%, B 0%, C 25%, D 0%, E 19%).

Table 1.3 The patterns of pigmentary demarcation lines are listed in the table below revised from James et al. [8]

A	Voigt's or Futcher's lines: anterior pectoral region and/or inner arms (hyperpigmented) (Fig. 1.13)
B	Posteromedial lower extremity (hyperpigmented)
C	Hypopigmentation of the central chest or abdomen vertically oriented over the pre- or para-sternal area (hypopigmented) (Fig. 1.14)
D	Posteromedial area of the spine (hyperpigmented) or curved convex line on face (hyperpigmented)
E	Line from mid-third of clavicle to the areola, bilaterally (hypopigmented) (Fig. 1.15)

Linea Nigra (Fig. 1.16)

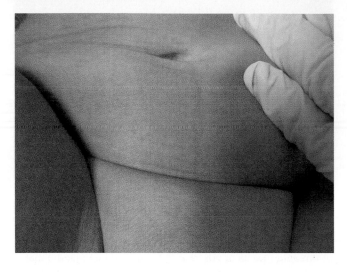

This photo demonstrates a fine linea nigra (Fig. 1.16) in a young child. Linea nigra is noted in 31.4% of children aged 0–15 years in Nigeria, increasing to 47.3% for children aged 16–30 years. Sex hormones are felt to increase the incidence, and pregnancy in particular, can cause the appearance of the linea nigra [9].

Periocular Hyperpigmentation (Fig. 1.17)

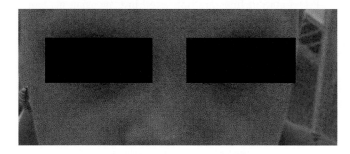

Periocular hyperpigmentation (Fig. 1.17) is observable in all races and is a combination of pigment from friction, ocular hypotensive agents, and dermatitis with vascular prominence through a thin periocular skin. In Caucasians, purple to red coloration from background vasculature is not uncommon, while brownish hyperpigmentation is seen in African Americans. In this Hispanic girl with atopic dermatitis and alopecia universalis, a hybrid of hyperpigmentation and violaceous tone are noted.

Hair Issues

Caucasian Hair Whorl (Fig. 1.18)

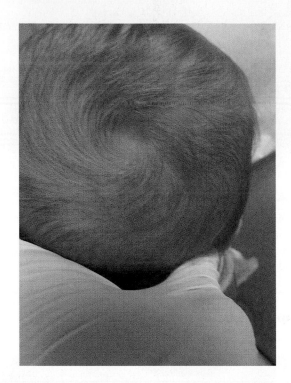

Hair whorls are best noted in straight-haired children especially Caucasian (Fig. 1.18) and Asian infants. Fine hair over the crown is common in Caucasian infants. Often, soft texture and thin caliber make for extra movement with light touch.

Asian Hair: Infant and Toddler (Figs. 1.19 and 1.20)

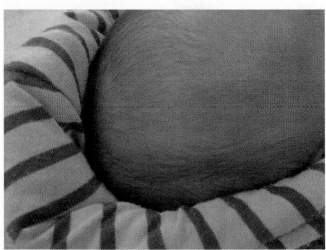

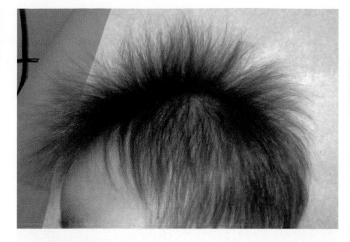

Hair of Black Child (Fig. 1.22)

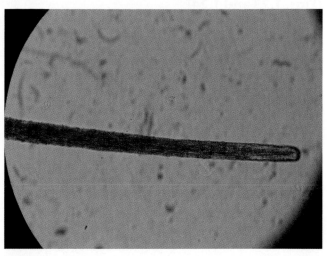

Asian infants have hairs of thin caliber extending over the forehead as vellus hairs (Fig. 1.19). Toddlers and pre-schoolers of South Asian descent demonstrate buoyancy of their hairs, allowing for the hairs to stand up on end without being touched (Fig. 1.20).

Microscopy of a Black child hair demonstrates discrete packets of pigment along the shaft as noted in Fig. 1.22 (Table 1.4).

Hispanic Hair Whorl (Fig. 1.21)

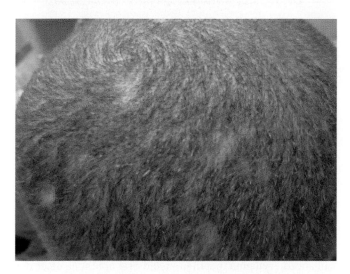

Table 1.4 Differences in hair [10]

Race	Hair morphology
Black (spiral) (in the United States: African American or Afro-Caribbean)	Flattened cross-section
	Textured hair
	Curved, helically shaped follicle
	Limited anchorage of follicles with elastic fibers
	Variable shaft diameters
	Lower hair density 0.6 follicular units per square millimeter
	Less water content than Caucasian hair
	Melanosomes in the outer root sheath and hair bulb
	Fewer elastic fibers anchoring hair follicles
Asian	Round cross-section
	Linear follicles
	Regular interfollicular spaces
	Hair density 1 follicular unit per square millimeter
Caucasian	Round to ovoid cross-section
	Linear to slightly curved follicles
	Variable interfollicular spaces
	Hair shaft diameters on the thighs and calves greater than in Black or Asian individuals
	Follicles are anchored with elastic fibers
	Hair density 1 follicular unit per square millimeter

Children of Hispanic or Latino descent may have straight to curly hair. In the straight-haired child, a hair whorl is observable. In a child whose hair favors that of Black children, an inability to note the hair whorl is expected. In the Hispanic child (Fig. 1.21), the presence of alopecia areata helps to highlight the natural whorled pattern, which might otherwise be obscured by curly hair.

Hyperpigmentation of the Scrotum
(Figs. 1.23 and 1.24)

Hyperpigmentation of the Gums
(Figs. 1.25 and 1.26)

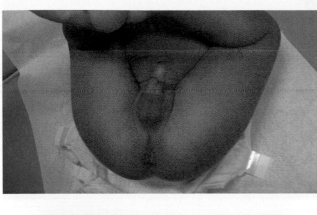

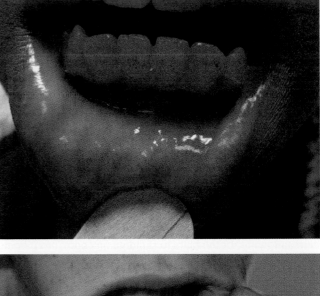

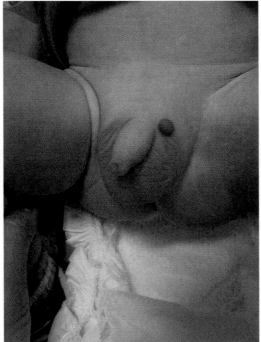

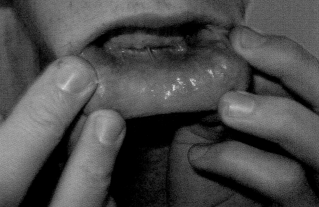

In the Hispanic infant in Fig. 1.23, pigmentation is notable over the scrotum and in the perianal area. Such pigmentation is notable at birth in most boys, but becomes more prominent as pigmentation develops in the first 6–12 months of life. The Caucasian infant in Fig. 1.24 also has slight hyperpigmentation to his scrotum due to thickened and rugose skin (Fig. 1.24). A juvenile xanthogranuloma is noted on his genitalia as well.

Gum hyperpigmentation can be a normal change with age in individuals of color, especially Black children (Fig. 1.25). Localized pigmentation can be noted in the gums as a nevoid phenomenon adjacent to a café au lait macule. This is in comparison to the light gums of a Caucasian child in Fig. 1.26, where pink coloration of the mucosa is noted. Enhanced erythema, papillation and oral aphthous ulcer due to contact dermatitis are also noted in Fig. 1.26. Excessive pigmentation of the gums can also be associated with Addison's disease, especially if very dark with abrupt onset. Further review of oral mucosal pigmentation can be found in Chap. 4 (Figs. 4.16 and 4.25).

References

1. http://www.whitehouse.gov/omb/fedreg_1997standards. Accessed 29 Nov 2011
2. http://www.hypertrichosis.com/hypertrichosis-causes/hairy-ears-elbows.shtml. Accessed 18 Dec 2011

3. Kelly AP (2009) Chapter 13: Nuances in skin of color. In: Kelly AP, Taylor SC (eds) Dermatology for skin of color. McGraw Hill, New York, pp 81–2

4. Taylor SC (2002) Skin of color: biology, structure, function, and implications for dermatologic disease. J Am Acad Dermatol 46 (2 suppl):S41–62

5. Nicolaides N, Rothman S (1952) Studies on the chemical composition of human hair fat: II, the overall composition with regard to age, sex and race. J Invest Dermatol 21:90

6. Kligman AM, Shelley WB (1958) An investigation of the biology of the sebaceous gland. J Invest Dermatol 30:99–125

7. Quatresooz P, Hermanns JF, Hermanns-Le T, Pierard GE, Nizet JL (2008) Laddering melanotic pattern of Langer's lines in skin of colour. Eur J Dermatol 18:575–8

8. James WD, Carter JM, Rodman OG (1987) Pigmentary demarcation lines: a population survey. J Am Acad Dermatol 16(3 Pt 1):584–90

9. George AO, Shittu OB, Enwerem E, Wachtel M, Kuti O (2005) The incidence of lower mid-trunk hyperpigmentation (linea nigra) is affected by sex hormone levels. J Natl Med Assoc 97(5):685–8

10. Heath CR, McMichael AJ (2009) Chapter 17: Biology of hair follicle. In: Kelly AP, Taylor SC (eds) Dermatology for skin of color. McGraw Hill, New York, pp 105–9

Neonatal Acne (Figs. 2.1–2.3)

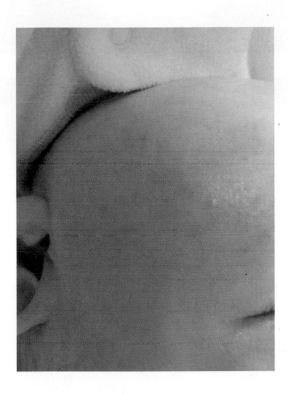

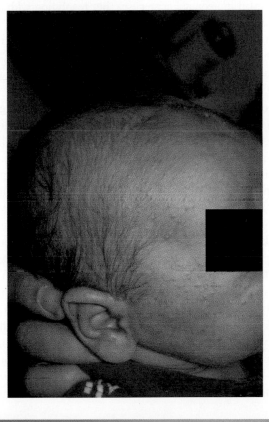

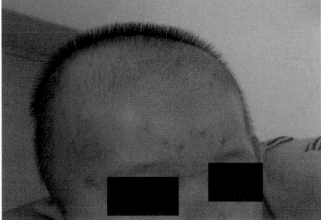

N.B. Silverberg, *Atlas of Pediatric Cutaneous Biodiversity: Comparative Dermatologic Atlas of Pediatric Skin of All Colors*,
DOI 10.1007/978-1-4614-3564-8_2, © Springer Science+Business Media, LLC 2012

Neonatal acne is a common disorder of infancy. In Caucasian children (Fig. 2.1), flesh-colored to pink monomorphic papules occur over the forehead and cheeks accompanied by few comedones. Neonatal acne is now felt to be at times due to inflammatory response to initial colonization with *Malassezia* species compounded by perinatal hormonal production and possibly transplacental hormonal transfers. *Malassezia* is often causative in cases along the hairline as would be seen in adolescence (Fig. 2.2). Rarely superficial candidiasis and group B *Streptococcus* can mimic acne and should be considered in widespread or atypical cases (invasive GBS is statistically more common in Black infants) [1]. Usage of gentle cleansing and topical antifungal or acne medicaments may be helpful in neonatal acne cases, but resolution with age is expected [2, 3].

In my personal observation, for Hispanic children and darker-skinned children, violaceous erythema can be associated with, and hyperpigmentation can be a result of neonatal acne, as would be noted in older patients (Fig. 2.3).

Acne occurs in every age group. In infants, acne is generally inflammatory in nature with notable follicular occlusion. Although acne can occur at any age, the presence of significant acne in prepubertal children outside of infancy should prompt examination for signs of virilization and for accelerated growth that might reflect androgen-secreting tumors or endocrinopathies such as congenital adrenal hyperplasia. Congenital adrenal hyperplasia is seen in Caucasian, Italian, Ashkenazi Jewish, Yupik Eskimo, Brazilian, Filipino, and Middle Eastern patients and rarely reported in Blacks [4]. While neonatal acne can persist, work-up for hyperandrogenism is warranted in children over the age of 1 year or in children with virilization or family history of congenital adrenal hyperplasia. As in older children, scarring is of concern in infantile acne. Although acne is treated similarly to adults in this age group, erythromycin orally replaces the usage of tetracyclines. Isotretinoin has been described as being effective in scarring cases, primarily in Caucasian children.

Perioral Dermatitis (Figs. 2.4–2.7)

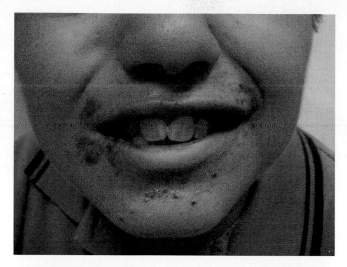

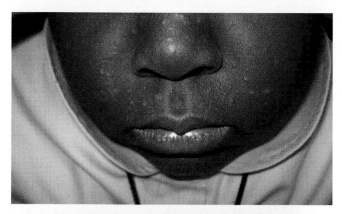

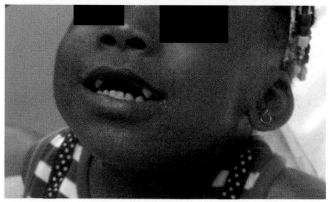

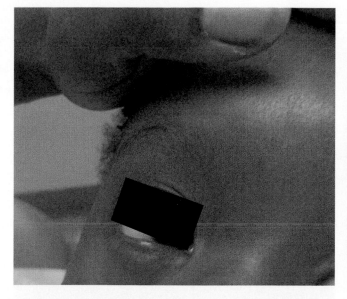

Preteen Acne (Figs. 2.8–2.11)

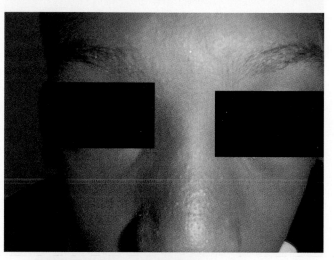

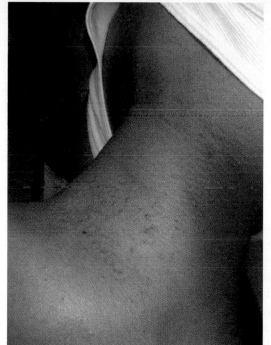

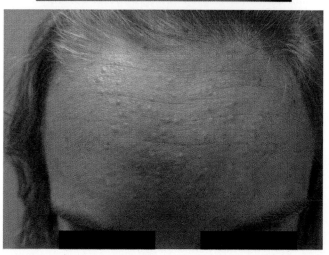

Perioral or periorificial dermatitis is a monomorphic papular acne that occurs in a periorificial distribution surrounding the eyes, nasal alae, and perioral regions. Genital involvement can occasionally be noted. Children with periorificial dermatitis often have atopic dermatitis. Lesions can be precipitated or flared by corticosteroid application (topical or inhalational) and/or by withdrawal of the same. Therapy with topical metronidazole, erythromycin and/or pimecrolimus or oral erythromycin (tetracycline for 9 years and over) is generally effective, but slow taper is needed after clearance to avoid withdrawal flares [5]. Lesions of periorificial dermatitis are more erythematous to flesh-toned in individuals who are Hispanic/Latino as noted in this 9-year-old Hispanic boy (Fig. 2.4) who had hydrocortisone 1% applied to his face prior to lesion onset.

Lesions of periorificial dermatitis in Black children are erythematous to flesh-toned (Fig. 2.5). Milder cases can have slightly hypopigmented papules (Fig. 2.5). More inflamed periorificial dermatitis in African American children can be more violaceous (Fig. 2.6) and may have associated background hyperpigmentation. Periorificial dermatitis is likely the same entity as the FACE (facial Afro-Caribbean childhood eruption) that has been described to be a granulomatous periorificial eruption [6]. This and infantile acropustulosis are the only forms of childhood acneiform diseases that are at least as common, if not more common, in children of color [7]. Ocular changes such as styes (hordeolum) and conjunctival erythema can be seen, similar to rosacea of adulthood (Fig. 2.7).

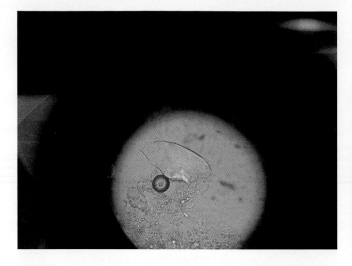

Pityrosporum Folliculitis of the Immunosuppressed (Fig. 2.12)

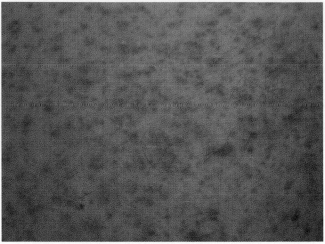

Preteen acne is often characterized by open and closed comedones and small papules over what is termed, the "T-zone" including the forehead and nasal bridge (Fig. 2.8). This type of acne is often amenable to medicated cleansers.

Early puberty has been noted in girls in the United States. Girls in the United States are in puberty by 7–8 years on average with Black and Hispanic girls entering puberty 6–12 months prior to Caucasian girls. A recent study noted that early puberty is likely the reason that children are seeking acne care earlier than they did 28 years ago, with Black girls having the earliest age of accessing acne care. The 6–8-year-old age group of children seems to be having the greatest relative increase in acne visits [8].

As noted in the African American patient in Fig. 2.8, prepubertal acne often manifests in Black children with flesh-colored papules.

In the pubescent years and thereafter, overgrowth of *Malassezia* species, which thrives on sebum, causes an inflammatory response termed seborrheic dermatitis. This yeast live off fats produced by the sebaceous glands, generally overgrowing on the scalp, face, neck, upper chest, back, and arms. Black children may have greater lipid content within sebum, driving this overgrowth [9, 10]. In preteens and younger teenagers, *Malassezia* overgrows in the hair follicle along with *Proprionobacterium acnes* [11]. The resultant appearance is monomorphic small papules, usually over the forehead, neck, and upper back.

In Fig. 2.9, a Hispanic teenager demonstrates lesions prominent over the neck region. This patient noted that he developed more lesions during football season, attributed to sweating and helmet usage. Papules are flesh-colored to violaceous. Figure 2.10 demonstrates a light-skinned Caucasian female who often wears bangs to cover, but accidentally exacerbates her pityrosporum folliculitis. Her potassium hydroxide preparation is shown in Fig. 2.11. While oral ketoconazole or fluconazole are effective, topical azole antifungals may be adequate therapy, but oral agents for acne are still required in many children [6].

In immunosuppressed individuals, pityrosporum folliculitis can be very extensive, as noted in this 15-year-old boy on chemotherapy (Fig. 2.12). In these cases, systemic therapy with oral antifungals is way more efficacious than topical agents.

Acne-Pomade Type (Figs. 2.13–2.15)

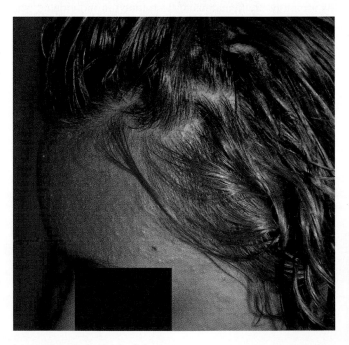

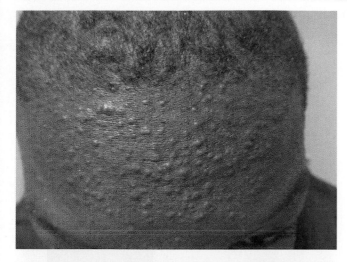

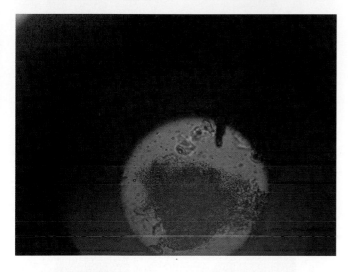

Acne with Postinflammatory Pigmentary Alteration (Figs. 2.16–2.18)

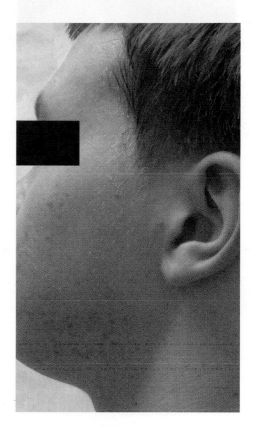

Pomade acne is caused by usage of hair pomades for styling than contain occlusive fats. This results in occlusion of the follicular units of the anterior scalp and forehead, producing hyperpigmented (in darker patients) to erythematous (in lighter skinned patients) monomorphic papules. This type of acne requires discontinuation of occlusive products and alteration to water or silicone-based hair products. Pomade acne is very common in Hispanic (Fig. 2.13) and Black teenagers due to hair styling trends in the former and drier hair shafts in the latter, requiring extra hydrating products [12].

In Fig. 2.14, the African American teenage boy demonstrates that pomade acne and pityrosporum folliculitis are often one and the same entity. Treatments to reduce *Malassezia* counts may benefit patients with pomade acne. In Fig. 2.15, potassium hydroxide 20% mixed with Swartz Lamkins stain highlights clusters of yeast in the superficial hair follicle consistent with pityrosporum folliculitis.

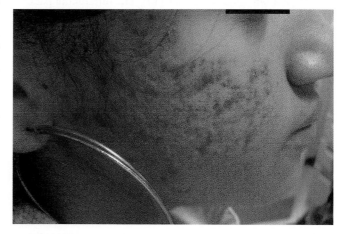

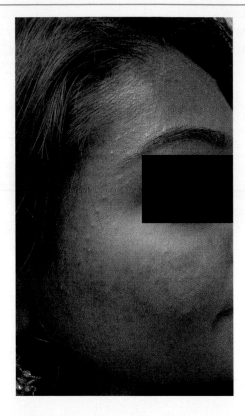

Indian (South Asian) teenager with acne vulgaris has enhancement of the features observed in Hispanic/Latino children, with greater prominence of hyperpigmentation and less prominent erythema due to obscuring by pigmentation.

Acne Before and After Isotretinoin Hispanic (Figs. 2.19 and 2.20)

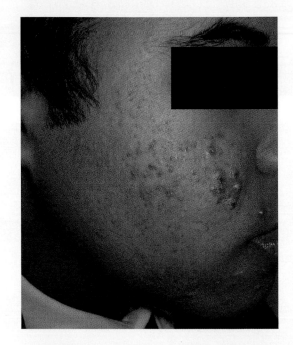

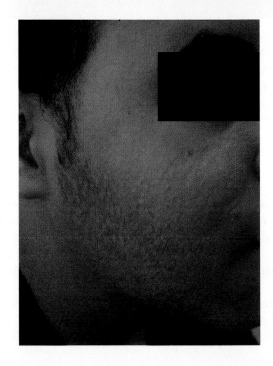

Acne vulgaris occurs in specific patterns in puberty that are consistently preserved irrespective of race, ethnicity, and social class. However, true nuances exist in the presentation of acne between races and ethnicity. In fact, in Black patients, hyperpigmentation and the postinflammatory sequelae of acne can be as or more likely to cause a patient to seek care than acne itself [13]. Some authors postulate that the hyperpigmentation noted in Black patients may relate to greater levels of inflammation in all acne lesions [14]. The differential patterns of dyspigmentation are the aim of the series of photographs.

Acne is typified in all individuals by five types of lesions: (1) the rudimentary precursor, the microcomedone, which is not visible to the naked eye, (2) the comedones, open and closed (blackheads and whiteheads) which are a result of follicular plugging (which may be caused by pro-inflammatory products of *P. acnes*, the bacterium that grows by feeding on sebum in the sebaceous follicle during puberty, (3) the papules and pustules that result from inflammation induced by *P. acnes*, (4) nodules, deeply inflamed and potentially ruptured follicles and (5) scarring-both temporary hyperpigmentation and scarring which may be of ice-pick, rolling or boxcar variants and/or keloids, especially noted as a type of scarring in Black individuals.

In the Caucasian teenager pictured in Fig. 2.16, erythema is noted where prior acne lesions had been. Acne vulgaris in Hispanic adolescents often has very prominent dyspigmentation, especially deep erythema, violaceous areas, and hyperpigmentation. The prominence of dyspigmentation creates a depth effect such that the skin appears more depressed or indented than it is in actuality (Fig. 2.17). In Fig. 2.18, the

Despite the presence of deep erythema and the perceptual appearance of depressed scars, this Hispanic 16-year-old male clears nearly fully, with limited sequelae after 5 months of isotretinoin dosed at 0.75–1 mg/g/day. Additionally, notable reduction in sebum production, albeit temporary, manifesting as reduced facial sheen, is noted in the post-therapy photo.

Acne Scarred (Fig. 2.21)

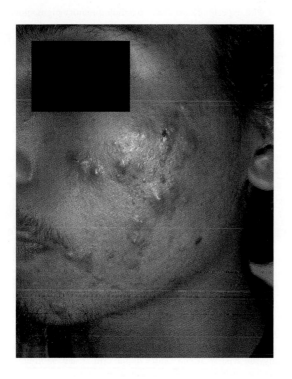

Cystic acne is equally common in Caucasians and Hispanics, but is less common in Asian and Black patients [15]. The 17-year-old Hispanic male in Fig. 2.21 has some of the important features of scarring acne, namely, extremely prominent erythema and nodules clustered over the hollow of the cheeks. He also demonstrates the rudiments of all three types of acne scars, ice pick scarring over the temples and the rudiments of rolling and/or boxcar scarring on the cheeks and chin area. While isotretinoin can reverse nodular lesions, persistent scarring may necessitate cosmesis using topical hydroquinones and retinoids, chemical peeling agents (e.g., glycolic acid), pulsed dye laser for erythema and hypertrophic scars and fractionated resurfacing laser for depressed scarring.

Hidradenitis Suppurativa (Fig. 2.22)

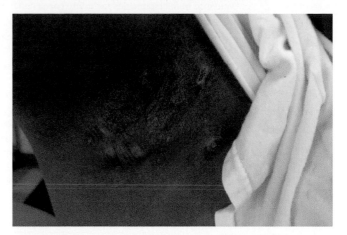

Cystic acne is associated with the follicular occlusion tetrad including: folliculitis decalvans, hidradenitis suppurativa (acne inversa), and pilonidal cysts. In the African American female noted in Fig. 2.22 we note some of the clinical features of Hidradenitis suppurativa including nodules, abscesses, fistulas (double comedones). Notable hyperpigmentation and violaceous hue are prominent in the nodules. When granulomatous changes are noted histologically, in hidradenitis suppurativa, most cases are caused by follicular foreign-body reactions, but consideration for the possibility of overlap with Crohn's disease (especially) in Caucasian children) and sarcoidosis (especially in Black children) should be given [16].

An association with increased body mass index may explain the presence of Hidradenitis suppurativa in obese teenagers [17]. Because the increasing prevalence of teen obesity is higher in individuals of color, this grouping may be particularly hard-hit by Hidradenitis suppurativa [18].

Oral tetracyclines or isotretinoin can aid medically, with axillary excision being the treatment with the most definitive clearance, but quite invasive. A new therapeutic option is photodynamic therapy; however, darker skin tones would be expected to have more risk of scarring after this procedure. There has been a report of squamous cell carcinoma in sites of chronic hidradenitis lesions of a Black individual, and this may be a racial association requiring closer lesional observation [19] (Table 2.1).

Table 2.1 Treatment for acne

Education	Dietary education includes low-glycemic index diet and avoidance of dairy
	Avoidance of thick pomades including cocoa butter, petrolatum, and unrefined mineral oil products on the face
	Use hair gels that are water-based or silicone-based
	Careful application of sunscreen each morning to minimize postinflammatory changes and to counteract drug-induced dryness or photosensitivity
	Avoidance of products recommended by nonprofessionals, e.g., toothpaste, baking soda, etc. as these enhance dyspigmentation
Medications	Topical medicaments (avoid high concentrations in individuals who experience extensive postinflammatory pigmentary alteration)
	Salicylic acid (0.5–2%)—Available in OTC therapies, this is comedolytic and enhances normal pigmentation
	Benzoyl peroxide—This medicament kills the pathogenic bacterium *P. acnes* by a nonantibiotic mechanism of killing, thereby reducing risk of oral and topical antibiotic resistance, while reducing active skin lesions
	Topical erythromycin or clindamycin—These topical antibiotics are also anti-inflammatory, but work synergistically in combination with benzoyl peroxide. Combination products often look white on dark patients and should be prescribed for after-school usage or at bedtime
	Topical dapsone—Anti-inflammatory agent that works through a nonantibiotic mechanism, thereby lacking risk of resistance (data for age 12 and over); effective in all skin tones, but reduces erythema well in Caucasian patients
	Topical azelaic acid—This agent is comedolytic and antibacterial, while also lightening hyperpigmentation; the product is useful for mild acne with excessive dyspigmentation and in women with sensitive facial skin
	Topical retinoids—These agents include prescription tretinoin, adapalene, and tazarotene. They are effective at clearing lesions and can be used as solo agents or in their compounded forms (e.g., tretinoin and clindamycin or adapalene and benzoyl peroxide)
Oral medications	Sub-antimicrobial doxycycline—Works by an anti-inflammatory mechanism with less gastrointestinal and phototoxicity side effects
	Oral tetracyclines—Minocycline, doxycycline, and tetracycline are all anti-inflammatory. Newer formulations with slow-release capsules can be given once-daily, improving compliance; not for usage for under age 9 years
	Oral erythromycin is reserved for oral usage in patients age 8 or under, or for tetracycline allergic individuals; stomach upset is not uncommon on this medication
	Oral trimethoprim-sulfamethoxazole or amoxicillin are reserved for patient with severe facial pustules who have cultures demonstrating gram negative bacteria, i.e., co-morbid gram negative folliculitis
	Oral isotretinoin—Anti-inflammatory, comedolytic and reduces sebum production, all of which contribute to less bacterial overgrowth. This drug is heavily regulated due to teratogenicity and reports of suicidality on the drug. Usage is limited to scarring acne or acne unresponsive to multiple courses (2+) of oral antibiotics, or to scarring acne
	Oral zinc supplementation has been described to reduce resistance to antibiotic agents
Cosmetic interventions: topical agents	Topical soybean trypsin inhibitor, contained in sunscreens reduces appearance of facial dyspigmentation
	Hydroquinones over the counter and prescription reduce appearance of hyperpigmentation
	Usage of calming agents may reduce facial flushing in Caucasian girls with combined acne vulgaris and acne rosacea (e.g., glycerrhetinic acid, feverfew)
Cosmetic interventions: procedures	Chemical peels using glycolic acid or salicylic acid can be performed safely if concentrations and times of exposure are increased gradually and conservatively; usage of hydroquinones in advance of the procedure reduces risk of adverse pigmentary changes
	Microdermabrasion can be used at lower settings on patients of all ages and skin types to enhance clearance of dyspigmentation
	Fractionated resurfacing lasers have been used in patients of color for reduction of dyspigmentation and acne scars
	Avoid dermabrasion, CO_2 laser and photodynamic therapy in patients of color as modalities of acne therapy

Minocycline-Induced Hyperpigmentation (Fig. 2.23)

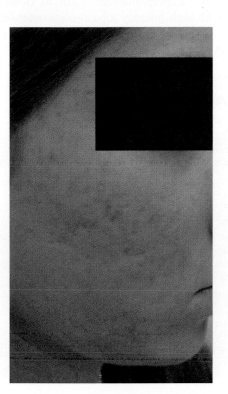

Minocycline is an anti-inflammatory tetracycline class antibiotic used for the treatment of acne vulgaris and Hidradenitis suppurativa. Dyspigmentation can occur with oral minocycline. Three types of minocycline-induced hyperpigmentation have been described: Type 1, blue-gray pigmentation in acne scars is shown in Fig. 2.23. Type II is blue-graying of the shins and forearms and Type III a diffuse muddy brown color of sun exposed areas. In this case, an aggressive facial at a department store had brought on the coloration acutely after 6 months of therapy with oral minocycline. In my experience, minocycline-induced hyperpigmentation is most obvious in Caucasian patients [20].

Steroid Acne (Fig. 2.24)

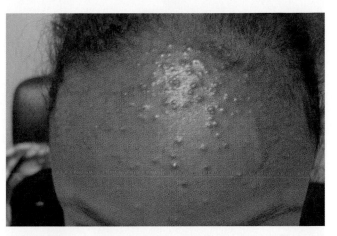

Steroid acne is a monomorphic, papulopustular acne occurring in the glabrous skin, caused by localized application of topical corticosteroids or via systemic ingestion of oral corticosteroids. This type of acne is similar to the appearance of monomorphic papular acne, being erythematous to flesh-colored papules in all races. The Hispanic teenage girl pictured in Fig. 2.24 developed acne along the hairline after application of topical corticosteroid solution in the hair for seborrheic dermatitis. Infrequent washing due to dryness of hair may promote seborrheic dermatitis in individuals of color. In the patient shown, potassium hydroxide preparation demonstrated yeast species, consistent with pityrosporum folliculitis. A single Korean study has supported the idea that steroid-induced acne may also be a form of pityrosporum folliculitis [21].

Infantile Acropustulosis (Figs. 2.25–2.27)

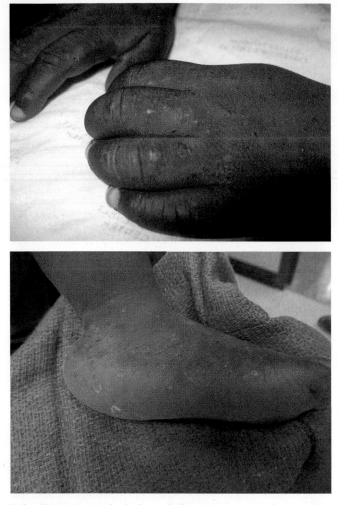

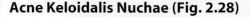

Flesh-colored to hyperpigmented pustules over the instep and plantar surface are here noted in the child in Fig. 2.27, who failed antiscabetic therapy. As can be noted, pustules appear to have hyperpigmentation due to violaceous tone. Therapy with high-potency topical corticosteroids and oral dapsone (1–2 mg/kg/day) can be effective, with monitoring for hemolysis in the latter.

Acne Keloidalis Nuchae (Fig. 2.28)

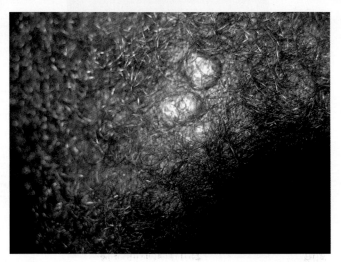

Acne Keloidalis Nuchae (Fig. 2.28) is a condition of individuals of color with curly hair who seek to style their hair by shaving the nuchal scalp. Shaving of this part of the scalp causes ingrown hairs, which in turn cause acneiform lesions and keloidal response [25]. Many of the acne kelo-idalis patients are obese and linkage to the metabolic syndrome has been noted, and in fact, this appears to be a risk factor for disease severity [26]. The teenage male in this picture required discontinuation of shaving of the nuchal scalp, topical antibiotics, and corticosteroids as well as intralesional triamcinolone for keloidal lesions. Patients who fail medical therapy may require surgical excision of the nuchal skin.

Infantile acropustulosis is an inflammatory pustular reaction noted in infancy through 3 years of age. In some series, increased prevalence in Black males is noted; however, all races and ethnicities may be affected at similar rates in larger studies [22]. In the Caucasian child in Fig. 2.25, small pustules appear flesh-colored to pink over the instep and extremities. Two out of three children with infantile acropustulosis have a preceding history of scabies. Initial presentation should prompt mineral oil preparation for scabies and when diagnosis of scabies is suspected or confirmed, antiscabetic therapy using 5% permethrin should be instituted. Because scabies is rampant in group facilities, international adoptees from Africa, South America, Asia, and Russia have been described with this condition as a postscabetic phenomenon [23]. Children in institutional care with palmar or plantar pustules should be presumed to have scabies, unless proven otherwise.

Lesions of acropustulosis occur over the distal extremities, especially the palms and soles, with recurrent crops of small papules and pustules (Fig. 2.26) that are intensely pruritic. Crops come every 2–4 weeks. Small pustules over the extremities can be noted in infantile acropustulosis. Potassium hydroxide preparation or a Wright stain of a pustule's contents will show neutrophils and eosinophils in fresh lesions [24].

References

1. Weston EJ, Pondo T, Lewis MM, Martell-Cleary P, Morin C, Jewell B et al (2011) The burden of invasive early-onset neonatal sepsis in the United States, 2005-2008. Pediatr Infect Dis J 30(11):937–941
2. Antoniou C, Dessinioti C, Stratigos AJ, Katsambas A (2009) Clinical and therapeutic approach to childhood acne: an update. Pediatr Dermatol 26:373–380
3. Davis EC, Callender VD (2010) A review of acne in ethnic skin: pathogenesis, clinical manifestations, and management strategies. J Clin Aesthet Dermatol 3(4):24–38
4. Therrell BL (2001) Newborn screening for congenital adrenal hyperplasia. Endocrinol Metab Clin North Am 30:15–30

5. Hall CS, Reichenberg J (2010) Evidence based review of perioral dermatitis therapy. G Ital Dermatol Venereol 145:433–444

6. Williams HC, Ashworth J, Pembroke AC, Breathnach SM (1990) FACE–facial Afro-Caribbean childhood eruption. Clin Exp Dermatol 15:163–166

7. Laude TA, Salvemini JN (1999) Perioral dermatitis in children. Semin Cutan Med Surg 18:206–209

8. Goldberg JL, Dabade TS, Davis SA, Feldman SR, Krowchuk DP, Fleischer AB (2011) Changing age of acne vulgaris visits: another sign of earlier puberty. Pediatr Dermatol 28(6):645–648

9. Nicolaides N, Rothman S (1952) Studies on the chemical composition of human hair fat: II, the overall composition with regard to age, sex and race. J Invest Dermatol 21:90

10. Kligman AM, Shelley WB (1958) An investigation of the biology of the sebaceous gland. J Invest Dermatol 30:99–125

11. Ayers K, Sweeney SM, Wiss K (2005) Pityrosporum folliculitis: diagnosis and management in 6 female adolescents with acne vulgaris. Arch Pediatr Adolesc Med 159:64–67

12. Laude TA (1995) Approach to dermatologic disorders in black children. Semin Dermatol 14:15–20

13. Alexis AF, Sergay AB, Taylor SC (2007) Common dermatologic disorders in skin of color: a comparative practice survey. Cutis 80:387–394

14. Halder RM, Holmes YC, Bridgeman-Shah S, Kligman AM (1996) A clinicohistopathologic study of acne vulgaris in black females (abstract). J Invest Dermatol 106:888

15. Taylor SC, Cook-Bolden F, Rahman Z et al (2002) Acne vulgaris in skin of color. J Am Acad Dermatol 46(2 suppl):S98–S106

16. Attanoos RL, Appleton MA, Hughes LE, Ansell ID, Douglas-Jones AG, Williams GT (1993) Granulomatous hidradenitis suppurativa and cutaneous Crohn's disease. Histopathology 23:111–115

17. Revuz JE, Canoui-Poitrine F, Wolkenstein P, Viallette C, Gabison G, Pouget F et al (2008) Prevalence and factors associated with hidradenitis suppurativa: results from two case control studies. J Am Acad Dermatol 59:596–601

18. Lee H, Lee D, Guo G, Harris KM (2011) Trends in body mass index in adolescence and young adulthood in the United States: 1959-2002. J Adolesc Health 49:601–608

19. Rosen T (1986) Squamous cell carcinoma: complication of chronic skin disorders in black patients. J Natl Med Assoc 78(12): 1203–1205

20. Geria AN, Tajirian AL, Kihiczak G, Schwartz RA (2009) Minocycline induced skin pigmentation: an update. Acta Dermatovenerol Croat 17:123–126

21. Yu HJ, Lee SK, Son SJ, Kim YS, Yang HY, Kim JH (1998) Steroid acne vs. Pityrosporum folliculitis: the incidence of Pityrosporum ovale and the effect of antifungal drugs in steroid acne. Int J Dermatol 37(10):772–777

22. Razera F, Olm GS, Bonamigo RR (2011) Neutrophilic dermatoses: part II. An Bras Dermatol 86:195–209

23. Good LM, Good TJ, High WA (2011) Infantile acropustulosis in internationally adopted children. J Am Acad Dermatol 65:763–771

24. Razera F, Olm GS, Bonamigo RR (2011) Neutrophilic dermatoses: part II. An Bras Dermatol 86:195–209

25. Shapero J, Shapero H (2011) Acne keloidalis nuchae is scar and keloid formation secondary to mechanically induced folliculitis. J Cutan Med Surg 15:238–240

26. Verma SB, Wollina U (2010) Acne keloidalis nuchae: another cutaneous symptom of metabolic syndrome, truncal obesity, and impending/overt diabetes mellitus? Am J Clin Dermatol 11:433–436

Introduction

Birthmarks can be localized, in a focal distribution, cover a body region (e.g., bathing suit nevus), or segmentally distributed along the Lines of Blaschko, developmental cutaneous embryonic segments; rarely birthmarks are generalized in nature.

There are three types of melanocytic nevi in childhood named by size as small (<1.5 cm), medium, or intermediate (>1.5 and <20 cm) and giant or large (20 cm or greater), the size being ultimate adult size. Although melanocytic nevi are noted at birth in up to 1.2–1.4% of Caucasian infants, acquisition of nevi, especially melanocytic nevi, occurs through the first 3–4 decades of life. In Caucasian children from Barcelona, ages 1–15 years, the average number of nevi is 17.5, 61.1% on the face and neck. Nevi increase in number steadily through childhood due to sun exposure, especially in individuals of light skin tone [1]; the average number of nevi at age 1 year is 1.5 (±2.1) and at 15 years 30.58 lesions (±22.64). Globular patterning accounts for about half of dermoscopic cases, followed by mixed reticular-globular and reticular alone. Globular pattern may be more common in lesions on the head, neck, and torso [2, 3].

Melanocytic Nevus-Blonde (Fig. 3.1)

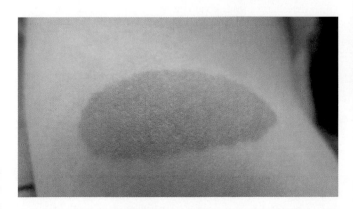

In lightly pigmented children of Fitzpatrick phototype I or II, who possess lightly pigmented hair, congenital melanocytic nevi (small <1.5 cm, medium >1.5 cm, and <20 cm^2) are often light tan in coloration during infancy. I term this the "blonde nevus," (Fig. 3.1) which will develop light colored hair while undergoing maturational changes of toddler and preschool years. The background skin pattern may also be indiscernible (homogenous) on handheld dermoscopy in fair-skinned individuals on dermoscopy early in childhood, or may have a faint reticular pattern as would be expected in pink nevi on the scalp [4, 5]. It is my personal observation that in many cases slight homogenous darkening of the nevus clinically, with improved pattern definition on dermoscopy, will occur in the first decade of life.

Eclipse Nevus (Figs. 3.2 and 3.3)

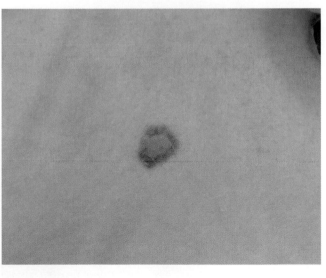

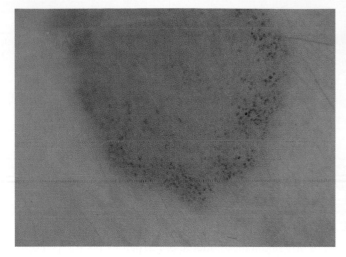

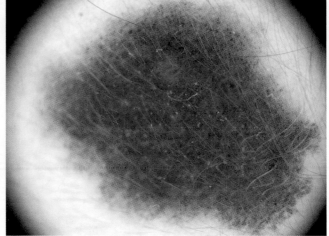

Red-heads and blondes may also develop the eclipse nevus (Fig. 3.2), where the center of the nevus is tan and the outer rim is more pigmented than the center [6]. Such nevi are commonly noted in glabrous skin, especially the scalp. Peripheral globular patterning [5] on dermoscopy can be noted in these lesions (Fig. 3.3).

Darker Nevi in Darker Children (Figs. 3.4–3.6)

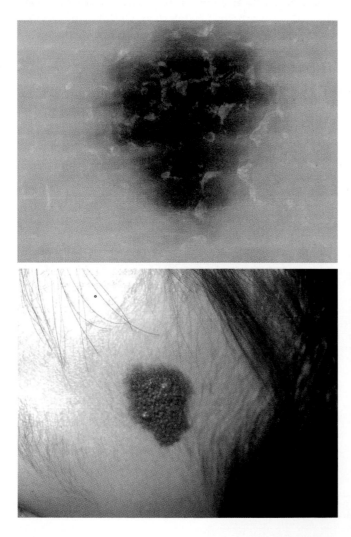

Children of Fitzpatrick phototype IV or greater who have darker hair may be born with or develop melanocytic nevi with darker brown pigmentation (Figs. 3.4 and 3.5).

Acquired melanocytic nevi of early childhood in darkly pigmented individuals often have a lighter rim (Fig. 3.6), especially noted with dermoscopy. Centrally, the pigment pattern can be quite dense making handheld dermoscopy difficult. Dermoscopic photographs may be easier to assess in these cases, as they remove the movement artifact noted in younger children and they allow for magnified review of the centrally darker portion. Irregularity, as in any individual, mandates observation, biopsy, and/or excision.

Plantar Nevus (Fig. 3.7)

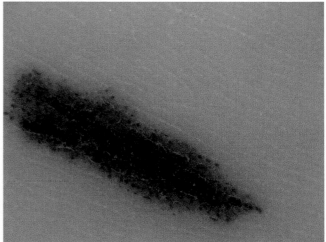

Acral melanocytic nevi are more common in Black (42%) than Caucasians (23%) in the United States, and the prevalence increases directly with skin pigmentation [7]. Nevi of the palms and soles often demonstrate pigmentary patterning along the dermatoglyphics of the skin (Fig. 3.7), resulting in parallel furrow patterns. In the palms and soles, one can see dermoscopically rows of pigmented globules (crista dotted/"peas in a pod" pattern) in a linear array to stripes of pigmentation (parallel furrow), most lesions demonstrating a hybrid of the patterns. Parallel ridge pattern requires close follow-up, as it can be seen in acral lentiginous melanomas [8]. In particular, close follow-up is needed in acral nevi in children of color due to higher incidence of acral lentiginous melanomas in individuals of color, this variant having a lower survival rate than melanomas overall at 5 and 10 years [9].

Maturation of the Medium-Sized Congenital Melanocytic Nevus (Fig. 3.8)

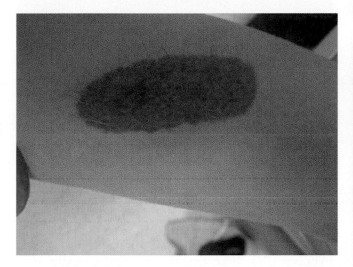

Clinically, maturational changes of the medium-sized congenital melanocytic nevus include homogenous thickening of nevus, slight papillation of the surface, increased pigmentation of "chocolate chips,"[1] small areas of darker appearance, and development of thick terminal hairs, usually of a slightly darker color and coarser texture than the scalp hair (Fig. 3.8). These changes are true whether the child is light- or dark-skinned.

Maturational changes in the congenital nevus begin in the toddler years and can progress until early puberty, but are usually stable in appearance by age 6 years. Congenital nevi will grow to be 2–3 times their original size over the course of the first 2 decades of life due to a stretch effect over the growing child. Clinically this is a 0.5–2 mm increase in size annually in most cases. More rapid increase in size should prompt biopsy.

---

[1] This terminology was taught to me by Annette Wagner, MD.

Dysplastic Nevus (Figs. 3.9 and 3.10)

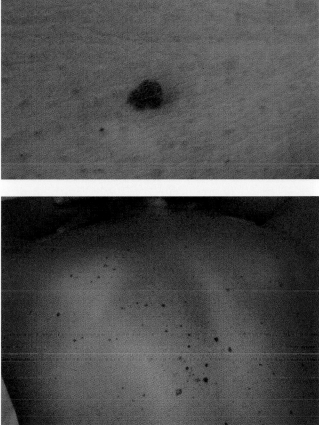

Caucasian children, especially those with a family history of dysplastic nevi or melanoma, children with a history of immunosuppression, and light-skinned children with a history of extensive photodamage will begin to develop dysplastic nevi (Figs. 3.9 and 3.10) in the prepubertal years.

These nevi have one or more alterations in the A (asymmetry), B (border irregularity), C (more than one color: red, white, or blue areas), D (diameter >6 mm), E (evolution) rules. Such nevi may or may not have a normally distributed pattern of pigmentation on dermoscopy. Many scalp melanocytic nevi in childhood display irregularity, even when the body melanocytic nevi do not. The reports of atypical scalp nevi seem to be primarily in light-skinned individuals [10]. Suspicion of melanoma should be high when lesions evolve rapidly, particularly when bleeding, ulceration, or appearance mimicking a pyogenic granuloma is noted. For this reason, it is best to remove all pyogenic granulomas of childhood by shave and electrodessication of the base in order to have a pathology specimen, and to avoid usage of topical agents such as imiquimod on suspected pyogenic granulomas [11]. Other suspicious features suggestive of melanoma can be noted on dermoscopy, including atypical pigment network, streaks, negative pigment network, chrysalis (white streaks), atypical dots and globules, irregular blotches, blue-white structures, atypical vascular structures, and peripheral brown structureless areas [3].

Dark Congenital Melanocytic Nevi of Children of Color (Fig. 3.11)

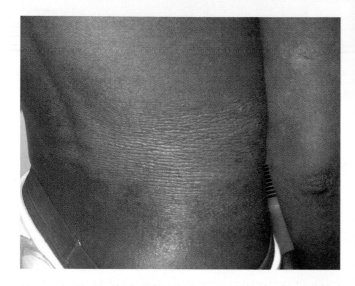

In darker Asian, Hispanic/Latino, or Black children (Fitzpatrick skin types IV–VI), congenital melanocytic nevi may be very dark brown (Fig. 3.11), bordering on black in coloration. These nevi have a globular or reticular pattern, central hyperpigmentation, and a dark brown coloration [12]. Dermoscopy with a dermoscopic camera attachment can aid in review of patterning in young children who tend to move during evaluation. Differentiation from areas of lichen simplex chronicus can be difficult at times and biopsy may be needed to confirm the melanocytic nature of the lesion.

Split Nevus (Figs. 3.12 and 3.13)

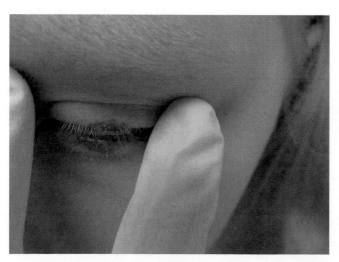

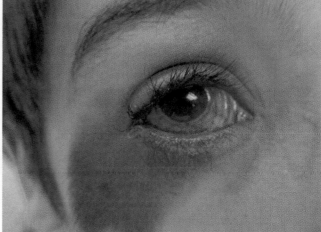

Split nevi (also known as divided nevi and kissing nevi) are congenital melanocytic nevi (splits can also occur with café au laits) that occur early on in utero prior to complete ocular, oral, or penile head development. In the case of the split ocular nevus, the lesion involves the upper and lower eyelids, and the mucosal surfaces. In my experience, the darker the individual, the more likely it is that the cornea/sclera will have visible pigmentation. In the Caucasian child (Fig. 3.12), the nevus is tan brown and the mucosal surface is minimally involved. In the split café au lait of the mouth, hyperpigmentation of the perioral skin and the adjacent mucosal surfaces including the gingiva are noted [13].

In the split nevus noted in the Arabic child (Fig. 3.13), the nevus is notably darker than that of a light Caucasian child and the nevoid pigmentation of the mucosa, the sclera, and cornea are more prominent in the darker patient.

Spitz Nevus (Fig. 3.14)

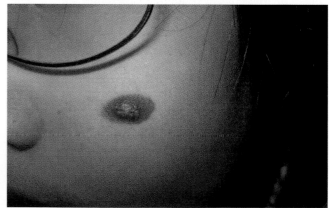

The Spitz nevus, once thought to be a juvenile melanoma, is a benign variant of acquired melanocytic nevus. In the Asian child in Fig. 3.14, light pink intonation to the Spitz nevus demonstrates the appearance of the Spitz nevus in Caucasian and Asian children. I have observed and/or seen case reports of Black children with Spitz nevi that may be black in color or resembling a pyogenic granuloma, prompting suspicion of melanoma; however, there are no published reports comparing the clinical appearance of Spitz nevi of childhood by race or ethnicity [14]. For this reason, therapy of pyogenic granulomas in childhood is best accomplished with shave and electrodessication rather than topical agents (e.g., imiquimod) [15]. Spitz nevi demonstrate specific patterns that are evenly distributed on dermoscopy including thick reticular, atypical globular, star burst, homogenous, negative pigment network, or atypical/multicomponent [3], the latter of which should be biopsied. Unless a clearly benign pattern is noted on dermoscopy, biopsy should be performed to rule out Spitzoid melanomas.

Café au lait Macule (Figs. 3.15–3.17)

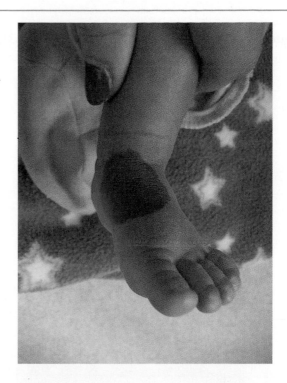

Café au lait macules are localized areas of hyperpigmentation which follow skin cleavage lines. These areas occur as a result of postzygotic gene mutations. Café au lait spots are hyperpigmented due to giant melanosomes or giant pigment granules and melanosome complexes around keratinocyte nuclei [16].

Six or more café au lait macules are the leading cutaneous marker of Neurofibromatosis type I [17]. Black children under the age of 5 years are statistically more likely to have one (22% vs. 11%) or two (5% vs. 2%) café au lait than Caucasian children [18]. However, Neurofibromatosis has no racial predilection.

Café au lait macules are generally 1–2 Fitzpatrick types darker than the natural skin tone. Café au lait macules (Fig. 3.15) and nevoid hypermelanosis often go unnoticed in lighter children until they become darker with age, possibly related to maturation of the pigment or in my opinion, enhanced due to sun exposure of the café au lait, tanning the area more so than the lighter natural skin tone.

Café au lait macules are noted within the first 3 months of life in children of Hispanic (Fig. 3.16) or Black descent and continue to become progressively more visible as pigmentation develops over the first 6–12 months of life.

Black children with café au lait macules (Fig. 3.17) have very obvious lesions at birth or within the first few months of life. The depth and darkness of pigmentation of these café au lait macules are often so dark that they suggest possible early nevus formation. Dermoscopy can aid in distinguishing these lesions, since the café au lait macule has no discernable pigment network.

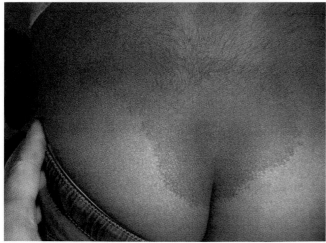

Neurofibromatosis Type I (Figs. 3.18 and 3.19)

Six or more such lesions of 5 mm or greater in childhood constitute one of the most consistent criteria for the diagnosis of neurofibromatosis type 1, a second criterion being required additionally. A pneumonic for the diagnostic criteria of neurofibromatosis type 1 is COLOR NF (Café au lait 6 or more 5 mm or greater in childhood, 1.5 cm or greater in adulthood); Optic glioma; Lisch nodules of the eyes; Osseous changes (e.g., sphenoid wing dysplasia or thinning of the long bone cortex without pseudarthrosis); relative with neurofibromatosis type I; neurological changes (seizures); freckling of the axillae or groin, i.e., Crowe's sign shown in Fig. 3.19 [20]. Café au lait lesions are generally 1–2 Fitzpatrick phototypes darker than the individual's natural skin tone (Fig. 3.18). However, darkening may occur with time. Café au lait macules may decrease in number with age after puberty in children with neurofibromatosis type I, inversely related to the increasing number of neurofibromas at puberty [21]. Multiple café au lait lesions may be associated with a variety of genetic syndromes. A single large café au lait, termed a Coast of Maine patch, can be noted in McCune Albright disease.

Pigmentary Mosaicism (Hypopigmented Type) (Fig. 3.20)

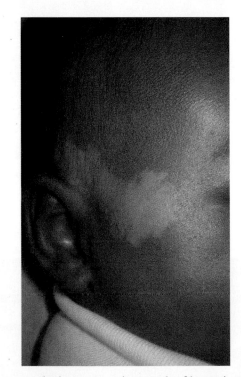

Nevoid pigmentary alterations may occur focally in ovoid areas of the skin or along the lines of Blaschko. Focal hyperpigmentation, termed a café au lait macule, is noted in about 2.83% of the normal pediatric population [19]. These lesions are due to localized increased pigment production in the absence of excess numbers of melanocytes.

The nevus depigmentosus is a patch of hypopigmentation with a ragged border that appears at birth in 50% and by 1 years of age in most patients [22]. The lesions, like café au lait spots, can be present on trunk, extremities or less commonly, head and neck. In the latter location, overlying blonde hairs (due to decreased eumelanin content) may be noted [23]. It can be distinguished from vitiligo vulgaris by not enhancing under Wood's lamp. In Asian patients hypopigmentation has been correlated to a reduction in the absolute number and more aggregation of melanosomes, as compared to normal surrounding skin. Single areas of pigmentary alteration of a nevoid nature are common in children of color. Multiple areas may warrant genetic work up for chromosomal abnormalities (e.g., chimerism), hypomelanosis of Ito (hypopigmented pigmentary mosaicism involving multiple segments of the skin), or tuberous sclerosis (ash leaf macules, confetti and thumbprint-like hypopigmentation).

Hypopigmented pigmentary mosaicism occurs in 0.4% of Asian newborns and will be noted in as many as 3% of Indian children [22]. Lesions can be focal, as in the lesion in Fig. 3.20 noted on the face in this African American infant.

In lighter skinned children, e.g., Caucasian or Asian children, hypopigmentation may not be notable until pigmentary development maturation by 6 months or until initial sun exposure of the affected area occurs, whereas half of all Indian children who have a nevus depigmentosus will have lesions visible at birth [22]. Although these lesions have been termed nevus depigmentosus, this is a misnomer. In fact, these are areas with melanocytes that produce pigment, although the amount of pigment is less than is normal for the individual. Patients with congenital pigmentary alterations are advised to use sun protection, as cumulative sun exposure appears to exacerbate the difference in pigmentation between normal and affected skin.

Twenty to thirty percent of children with multiple areas of hypopigmentation along the lines of Blaschko will have Hypomelanosis of Ito, a constellation of pigmentary mosaicism and developmental delay.

Nevus Depigmentosus Wood's Lamp Negative (Fig. 3.21)

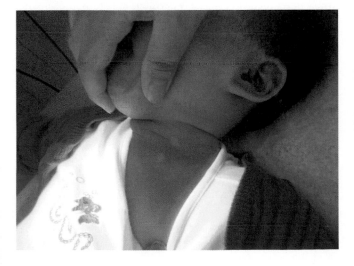

In Fig. 3.21 an Asian infant is featured who has an area of hypopigmented pigmentary mosaicism that is negative for enhancement with Wood's lamp due to the presence of active pigment production.

Nevus of Ota (Figs. 3.22–3.24)

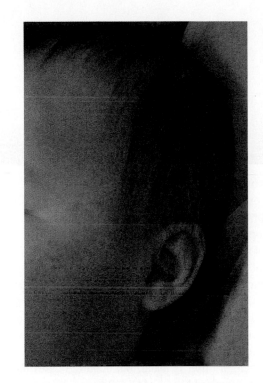

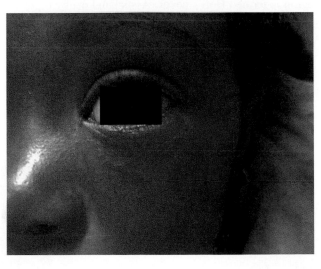

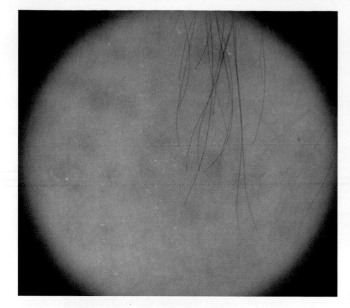

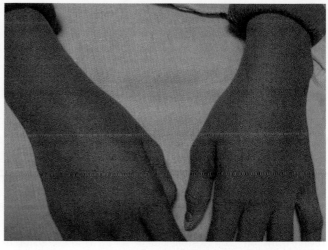

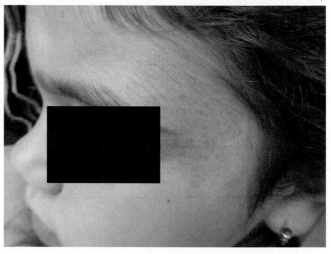

Nevus of Ito (when ocular changes are absent and lesions are noted over the lower face V3 trigeminal distribution, neck, and upper shoulders) and Nevus of Ota (Nevus fusco-caeruleus ophthalmo-maxillaris over the V1 and V2 distribution and associated with conjunctival pigmentation) are localized areas of dermal melanocytes in the dermis. The bluish discoloration is a result of the Tyndall effect. Pigmentation can vary from deep brown to blue. The lesion is more common in Asian (Fig. 3.22) and less so in Black children (Fig. 3.23). The second child demonstrates the dermoscopy without a patterned appearance of pigmentation (Fig. 3.24).

Congenital onset is usual, but acquired cases have been reported. Acquired Nevus of Ota like macules over the malar region is termed Hori's nevus. Associated ocular pigmentation can be noted in this African American girl (Fig. 3.23). Ocular pigmentation appears more commonly in darker individuals with this nevus [24]. Treatment using an NdYag 1,064 nm laser has been described.

Acral Lentiginosis (Figs. 3.25–3.27)

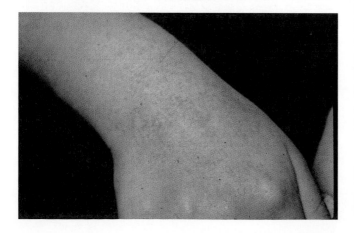

Acral lentiginosis is a form of clustered ephelides overlying the wrists/dorsal hands (Fig. 3.25) and ankles/dorsal feet. This form of pigmentation can be noted in all skin types, but is more notable in individuals of color, especially Indians (Fig. 3.26) and African Americans. Concurrent lentiginous pigmentation is not uncommon in other areas, but does not affect the mucosal surfaces. One such area is the periocular region (Fig. 3.27). Other sites I have noted in my practice include central chest and extension up the forearms; however, these areas are always clustered lentigines within a well-demarcated area and are usually symmetric. Areas of acral lentiginosis are extremely well demarcated over the wrist, as opposed to the widespread lentigines seen in Carney complex, Peutz–Jeghers syndrome, and LEOPARD syndrome. Furthermore, internal findings are lacking with acral lentiginosis.

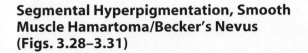

Segmental Hyperpigmentation, Smooth Muscle Hamartoma/Becker's Nevus (Figs. 3.28–3.31)

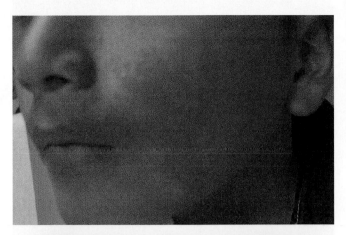

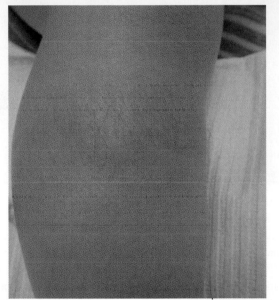

Nevoid hypermelanosis (Fig. 3.28) localized broadly in a segmental distribution (checkerboard) may have ill-defined borders, unlike the café au lait. This form of pigmentary alteration can be seen overlying a dermal nevoid process, such as a Becker's nevus, which is a late-onset epidermal nevus of smooth muscle, with overlying pigmentation and hypertrichosis. Congenital onset of a similar lesion is termed a smooth muscle hamartoma. A smooth muscle hamartoma is a congenital hamartoma which combines nevoid hypermelanosis, excess smooth muscle, and sometimes excess hair.

Becker's nevi are generally seen over the shoulder or hip girdle in preteens and teenagers. Hormonal receptors (e.g., estrogen) may account for appearance at puberty. Although of late onset, Becker's nevi can be associated (in 23%) with anomalies and/or tumors arising in the nevus, including accessory areola, underlying soft tissue (e.g., breast hypoplasia), vascular, bony or neural anomalies (Becker's nevus syndrome), and rare case reports of desmoid tumor, liposarcoma and melanoma. Therefore, patients should be instructed to return for any alterations arising in the texture or coloration of the nevus [25]. An acronym for the features of the Becker's nevus syndrome on the face is HATS (hemi maxillary enlargement, asymmetry of face, tooth abnormalities, and skin findings) [26].

In a Caucasian child, the background café au lait of a smooth muscle hamartoma or a Becker's nevus may be subtle (Fig. 3.29) as opposed to a Hispanic child (Fig. 3.30). In the African American patient in Fig. 3.31 dark background coloration allows for more defined borders.

In general, the hair is more obvious in darker children who have thick or curly body hair, making the diagnosis, but not the entity, more common in some children of color. The same is true for men vs. women, i.e., the diagnosis is easier in males due to greater body hair and more prominent hypertrichosis.

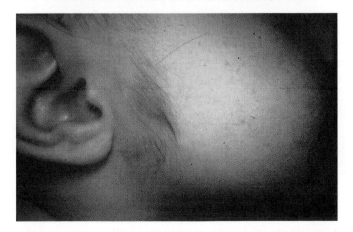

Nevus Sebaceus (Figs. 3.32–3.36)

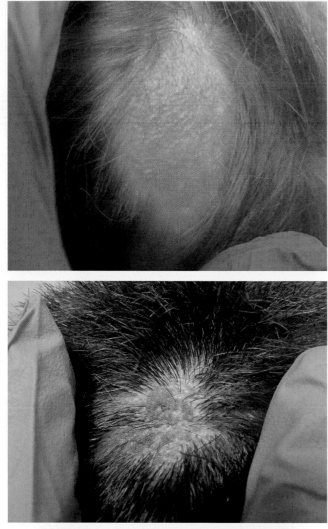

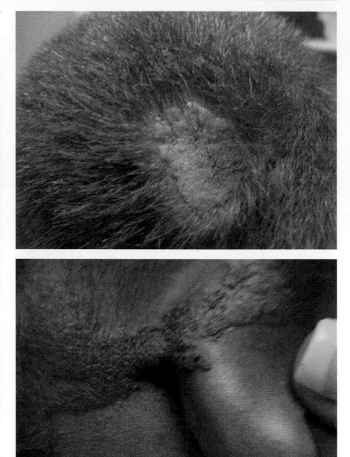

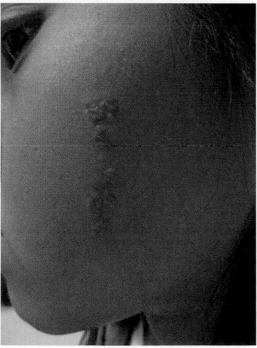

The nevus sebaceus of Jadassohn is an epidermal nevus of the skin of the scalp or face that contains excessive sebaceous glands. Histologically, such glands are rudimentary in infancy and become more enlarged with age. In infancy overlying seborrheic dermatitis can localize to the nevus sebaceus [27]. In prepubertal children the nevus sebaceus is a benign nevus. However, at puberty these lesions may develop thickening and rugose appearance, benign tumoral changes such as trichoblastomas and syringocystadenoma papilliferum or malignant changes including basal cell carcinomas, squamous cell carcinomas, and a variety of adnexal tumors. Tumors are primarily noted in nevus sebaceus of the scalp. In Caucasians, the nevus sebaceus is orange-yellow in color (Fig. 3.32). Benign thickening and verrucous surface changes with a preservation of the pink-yellow coloration are typical of pubertal alterations in a Caucasian nevus sebaceus (Fig. 3.33).

The nevus sebaceus is also orange-yellow as seen on the face of the Asian teenager in Fig. 3.34. One can note thickening that would be consistent with early pubertal thickening. Observation for malignant changes is often easier in facial nevus sebaceus, especially as the rate of tumor formation appears less common for the face as compared to the scalp.

In the Hispanic child in Fig. 3.35, the nevus sebaceus is of a brown skin tone, obscuring yellow-orange coloration of the sebaceous glands. These early verrucous changes are light, but can darken with age, further obfuscating observation for skin cancers.

In the nevus sebaceus in a darkly pigmented African American child in Fig. 3.36, orange-yellow appearance is not noted. As would be expected for darker Hispanic, Indian, and African American children with nevus sebaceus, the lesion is dark tan to dark brown without orange-red undertones. Rugose thickening and irregular surface changes of maturation can obscure detection of skin cancers, necessitating excision in these patients. In my experience, the surface elevations are usually larger in individuals of color than the filiform projections noted in Caucasian nevus sebaceus of puberty; however, there are no head to head longitudinal studies comparing appearance and tumor formation by race and/or ethnicity.

Flattening of lesions can be accomplished through a variety of topical agents including retinoids, which worked in this child, 5-flourouracil, imiquimod 5%, or chemical peeling agents. Resurfacing laser, pulsed dye laser, and electrodessication of the base can make lesions flatter and less noticeable without eliminating cancer risk, but the latter did not benefit this patient. As the facial lesions are not as verrucous and have fewer propensities to carcinomatous changes of the nevus, observation without excision is generally done for facial nevus sebaceus.

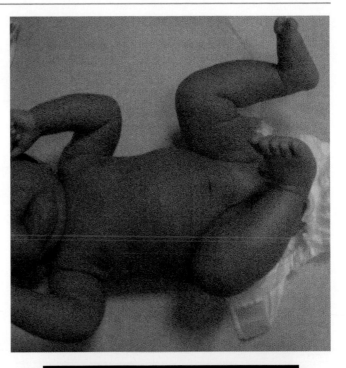

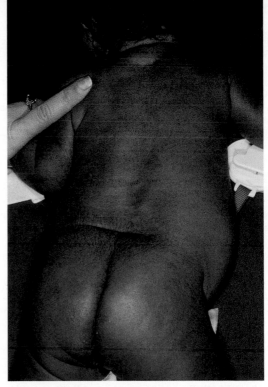

Mongolian Spot (Figs. 3.37–3.39)

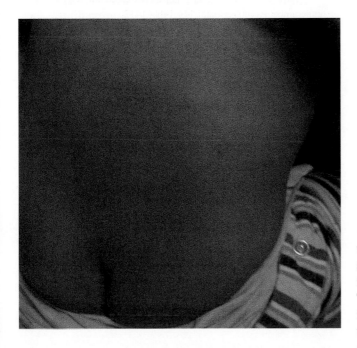

The Mongolian spot is a benign temporary pigmentation, usually of infants 2,500 g or greater in weight, that represents melanocytes in the dermis, the color of which, when filtered through the skin, produces a bluish color through the Tyndall effect. Lesions are usually present at birth or in the first few weeks of life. Lesions are most commonly noted in the sacral and gluteal areas (Fig. 3.37) [28]. The Mongolian spot is seen in less than 9.5–18.9% of Caucasian infants,

46% of Hispanic/Latino, 62.2% of Indian [29], 83.6% of Asian, and 96% of Black newborns [30, 31].

In Fig. 3.38, one can note eccentric lesions over the chest, abdomen, and extremities, notably sparing the umbilicus and breast tissue. On the extremities, lesions will be noted over the extensor surfaces. Resolution over the first few years of life is typical and nearly universal by age 6 years.

The Mongolian spot is deeper blue due to background skin pigmentation in the African American infant (Fig. 3.39). Eccentric lesions are here noted over the axial skin of the back and shoulder girdles, the latter being the second most common site. Like the primary lesions of the sacral Mongolian spot, the eccentric locations are more common in children of color. However, very extensive lesions can be associated with the mucopolysaccharidoses, such as Hunter's or Hurler's disease [32, 33].

Acknowledgments Many thanks to Dr. Ashfaq Marghoob for his interesting and expert insight into melanocytic nevi of childhood.

References

1. Vallarelli AF, Harrison SL, Souza EM (2010) Melanocytic nevi in a Brazilian community of predominantly Dutch descent (1999-2007). An Bras Dermatol 85:469–477
2. Aguilera P, Puig S, Guilabert A, Julià M, Romero D, Vicente A, González-Enseñat MA, Malvehy J (2009) Prevalence study of nevi in children from Barcelona. Dermoscopy, constitutional and environmental factors. Dermatology 218:203–214
3. Haliasos HC, Zalaudek I, Malvehy J, Lanschuetzer C, Hinter H, Hofmann-Wellenhof BR, Marghoob AA (2010) Dermsocopy of benign and malignant neoplasms in the pediatric population. Semin Cutan Med Surg 29:218–231
4. Scope A, Marghoob AA, Chen CS, Lieb JA, Weinstock MA, Halpern AC, SONIC Study Group (2009) Dermoscopic patterns and subclinical melanocytic nests in normal-appearing skin. Br J Dermatol 160:1318–1321
5. Tcheung WJ, Bellet JS, Prose NS, Cyr DD, Nelson KC (2011) Clinical and dermoscopic features of 88 scalp naevi in 39 children. Br J Dermatol 165:137–143
6. Schaffer JV, Glusac EJ, Bolognia JL (2001) The eclipse naevus: tan centre with stellate brown rim. Br J Dermatol 145:1023–1026
7. Palicka GA, Rhodes AR (2010) Acral melanocytic nevi: prevalence and distribution of gross morphologic features in white and black adults. Arch Dermatol 146:1085–1094
8. Minagawa A, Koga H, Saida T (2011) Dermoscopic characteristics of congenital melanocytic nevi affecting acral volar skin. Arch Dermatol 147:809–813
9. Bradford PT, Goldstein AM, McMaster ML, Tucker MA (2009) Acral lentiginous melanoma: incidence and survival patterns in the United States, 1986-2005. Arch Dermatol 145:427–434
10. Gupta M, Berk DR, Gray C, Cornelius LA, Bayliss SJ (2010) Morphologic features and natural history of scalp nevi in children. Arch Dermatol 146:506–511
11. Roldán FA, Hernando AB, Cuadrado A, Blanco CC, Fernández RS, Hermosa JM, Ochaita PL (2009) Small and medium-sized congeni-

tal nevi in children: a comparison of the costs of excision and long-term follow-up. Dermatol Surg 35:1867–1872
12. Zalaudek I, Argenziano G, Mordente I, Moscarella E, Corona R, Sera F, Blum A, Cabo H, Di Stefani A, Hofmann-Wellenhof R, Johr R, Langford D, Malvehy J, Kolm I, Sgambato A, Puig S, Soyer HP, Kerl H (2007) Nevus type in dermoscopy is related to skin type in white persons. Arch Dermatol 143:351–356
13. Sergay A, Silverberg NB (2007) Divided café-au-lait macule of the mouth. J Am Acad Dermatol 56:S98–S99
14. Carr EM, Heilman E, Prose NS (1990) Spitz nevi in black children. J Am Acad Dermatol 23:842–845
15. Tritton SM, Smith S, Wong LC, Zagarella S, Fischer G (2009) Pyogenic granuloma in ten children treated with topical imiquimod. Pediatr Dermatol 26:269–272
16. Takahasi M (1976) Studies on café au lait spots in neurofibromatosis and pigmented macules of nevus spilus. Tohoku J Exp Med 118:255–273
17. Nunley KS, Gao F, Albers AC, Bayliss SJ, Gutmann DH (2009) Predictive value of café au lait macules at initial consultation in the diagnosis of neurofibromatosis type 1. Arch Dermatol 145:883–887
18. Whitehouse D (1966) Diagnostic value of the café-au-lait spot in children. Arch Dis Child 41:316–319
19. Karabiber H, Sasmaz S, Turanli G, Yakinci C (2002) Prevalence of hypopigmented maculae and café-au-lait spots in idiopathic epileptic and healthy children. J Child Neurol 17:57–59
20. Ferner RE (2010) The neurofibromatoses. Pract Neurol 10:82–93
21. Duong TA, Bastuji-Garin S, Valeyrie-Allanore L, Sbidian E, Ferkal S, Wolkenstein P (2011) Evolving pattern with age of cutaneous signs in neurofibromatosis type 1: a cross-sectional study of 728 patients. Dermatology 222:269–273
22. Dhar S, Kanwar AJ, Kaur S (1993) Nevus depigmentosus in India: experience with 50 patients. Pediatr Dermatol 10:299–300
23. Fukai K, Ishii M, Kadoya A, Hamada T, Wakamatsu K, Ito S (1993) Nevus depigmentosus systematicus with partial yellow scalp hair due to selective suppression of eumelanogenesis. Pediatr Dermatol 10:205–208
24. Mishima Y, Mevorah B (1961) Nevus Ota and nevus Ito in American Negroes. J Invest Dermatol 36:133–154
25. Sciallis GF, Sciallis AP (2010) Becker nevus with an underlying desmoid tumor: a case report and review including Mayo Clinic's experience. Arch Dermatol 146:1408–1412
26. Happle R (2010) The group of epidermal nevus syndromes. Part I. Well defined phenotypes. J Am Acad Dermatol 63:1–22
27. Heilig S, Koslosky K, Ioffreda MD, Shin HT, Zaenglein AL (2011) Eczematous nevus sebaceus: a report of three cases. Pediatr Dermatol 28:176–179
28. Reza AM, Farahnaz GZ, Hamideh S, Alinaghi SA, Saeed Z, Mostafa H (2010) Incidence of Mongolian spots and its common sites at two university hospitals in Tehran, Iran. Pediatr Dermatol 27:397–398
29. Nanda A, Kaur S, Bhakoo ON, Dhall K (1989) Survey of cutaneous lesions in Indian newborns. Pediatr Dermatol 6:39–42
30. Cordova A (1981) The Mongolian spot: a study of ethnic differences and a literature review. Clin Pediatr (Phila) 20:714–719
31. Monteagudo B, Labandeira J, León-Muiños E, Carballeira I, Corrales A, Cabanillas M, Suárez-Amor O, Toribio J (2011) Prevalence of birthmarks and transient skin lesions in 1,000 Spanish newborns. Actas Dermosifiliogr 102:264–269
32. Rybojad M, Moraillon I, Ogier de Baulny H, Prigent F, Morel P (1999) Extensive Mongolian spot related to Hurler disease. Ann Dermatol Venereol 126:35–37
33. Ochiai T, Ito K, Okada T, Chin M, Shichino H, Mugishima H (2003) Significance of extensive Mongolian spots in Hunter's syndrome. Br J Dermatol 148:1173–1178

Melanonychia Striata Hispanic (Fig. 4.1)

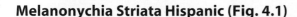

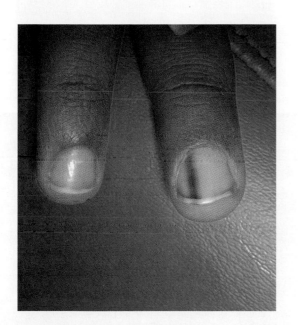

Melanonychia striata (Fig. 4.1) is a vertically-oriented linear hyperpigmentation of the nails, which results from excess pigment production in the nail matrix, which then moves along the grooves of the nail bed as the nails grow. This can be a benign phenomenon related to trauma in individuals of color. Medications may promote nail hyperpigmentation. Congenital nevi of the nail unit can present similarly. Usually such nevi have normal dermoscopic findings. Due to the rarity of melanonychia striata in Caucasian and Asian children, the likelihood is that linear pigmented lesions under the age of 20 years are melanocytic proliferations, rather than hyperpigmentation [1].

Laugier-Hunziker (Fig. 4.2)

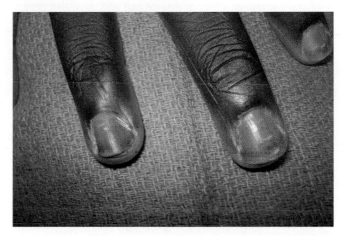

Melanonychia striata is seen in children of color, especially Black and Hispanic children. Seven percent of adult Blacks will have melanonychia, compared to 11.4% of Japanese and almost no whites. Melanocytes in Japanese patients have both immature and mature melanosomes, while Black patients have mature and dense melanosomes of the nail matrix [2]. However, individuals of color, though they have a lower incidence of melanoma than Caucasians, will proportionally have more acral melanomas than lighter individuals. Hence, observation and monitoring of pigmented lesions of the nail bed in children of color is required.

A condition in which benign pigmentation occurs in the oral mucosa and digits is termed Laugier-Hunziker. In these individuals, pigmentation of the gums and lips (lentigines) and melanonychia striata (Fig. 4.2) can be seen. Other forms of traumatic pigmentation in these patients include oral papillary hyperpigmentation and pinpoint pigmentation of the fingertips at the free margin of the nail. Skin manifestations of Laugier-Hunziker are nearly identical to Peutz–Jeghers syndrome, a cancer syndrome

N.B. Silverberg, *Atlas of Pediatric Cutaneous Biodiversity: Comparative Dermatologic Atlas of Pediatric Skin of All Colors*, DOI 10.1007/978-1-4614-3564-8_4, © Springer Science+Business Media, LLC 2012

Table 4.1 Features of pigmented nail lesions that may warrant nail bed biopsy [21]

Dark lesions—black or dark brown
Broad lesion (>5 mm)
Changing lesion
Hutchinson's sign (extension of pigmentation of the proximal nail fold)
Irregular dermoscopic patterning
Overlapping presence of subungual vascular lesions, especially pyogenic granuloma-like lesions
Paronychial hyperpigmentation isolated to same nail in the absence of other nails
Solitary lesion
Variegated lesion (especially new black, red, white, or blue changes)

in which polyposis and colon cancers is noted. Children with melanonychia striata and typical oral mucosal pigmentation require gastrointestinal work-up for polyposis [3].

Acral melanoma of the matrix or nail unit may also present with linear hyperpigmentation of the nail. Acral melanomas are a common presentation of melanoma in the uncommonly affected patient of color. Table 4.1 reviews some of the important clinical features that discern malignant and benign lesions of the nail unit. Dermoscopy of the pigmented lesion over the nail and dermoscopy of the pigmentation at the free margin of the nail should reveal pigmentary findings similar to those of nevi of the palms and soles, i.e., pigmentation following the grooves, the vertical pattern of the dermal papillae in the nail bed under the nail. When disorganization is noted, melanoma is suggested [4].

Pseudo-Hutchinson's Sign (Fig. 4.3)

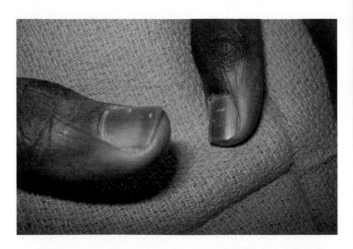

Many individuals of color, particularly children with xerosis and atopic dermatitis will have hyperpigmentation of the nail bed and matrix which reflects through the paronychial fold as hyperpigmentation (Fig. 4.3). In these benign cases, hyperpigmentation is usually light, evenly distributed across many nails, and with no alteration in relation to pigmented nail bands. The cuticles will not be hyperpigmented in such cases, since the pigment is from a deeper source.

Vitiligo (Figs. 4.4 and 4.5)

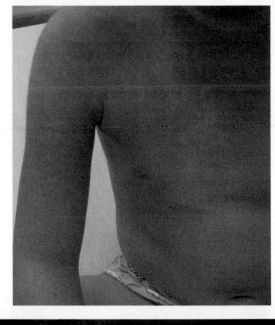

Vitiligo vulgaris is a disorder in which the body loses melanocytes and pigmentation (Table 4.2). Worldwide incidence is similar in all populations at 0.4–1%, except for a solitary Indian region where disease is noted to be as high as 8.8% [5]. Autoimmune attack of pigment cells occurs due to antibody production, derangements in B and T cell activity allowing for attack of self, alterations in pigment genes, alterations in genes participating in innate immunity, and aggravated oxidative destruction of pigment cells [6]. Association with other forms of autoimmunity in the patient and in second and first degree relatives is often noted. Autoimmune attack may injure, reduce function or trigger cell death of melanocytes. Vitiligo may be localized and the segmental type is common in childhood. Generalized types

Table 4.2 Work-up for individuals with generalized vitiligo

Physical examination for typical appearance and location
At onset of disease, full body examination for atypical melanocytic lesions that may have triggered disease onset (rare)
Wood's lamp examination
Biopsy for hematoxyllin and eosin and melanin stains where clinical disease is atypical
For confirmed cases, laboratory testing can be performed
Complete blood count, complete metabolic profile, thyroid function screen and 25 (OH) Vitamin D
Optional antithyroglobulin and antithyroid peroxidase antibodies
When phototherapy is planned: or expected antinuclear antibody to identify subjects who will have phototoxic reactions at low dosages of ultraviolet therapy and as baseline before psoralens and UV therapy which can induce antinuclear antibody formation.
Optional testing: Homocysteine (marker of severity), Vitamins B6, B12, and Folate (potentially reduced in vitiligo patients, especially South American and Indian (vegetarian) patients)

often affect the periorificial, intertriginous regions, and the skin over joints or bony prominences [2].

The Wood's lamp is a handheld UVA light source, emitting at 365 nm, which causes enhancement or increased prominence of vitiligo lesions as shown in Figs. 4.4 and 4.5. The reason for the enhancement has been posited to be either dermal reflectance of UV light or reflectance by tetrahydrobiopterin pathway by-products released in the inflammatory process. The Wood's lamp cannot rule out mycosis fungoides, as hypopigmented mycosis fungoides may similarly enhance [7].

For individuals with an olive or intermediate skin tone, including Hispanic and Indian patients, gradations of color loss can be noted in their vitiliginous lesions, termed trichrome vitiligo (Fig. 4.6). Areas of partial pigmentation in this condition, have greater numbers of pigment cells (albeit poorly functioning), thereby responding preferentially well (more rapidly) to ultraviolet light treatments [8].

Vitiligo-Speckled Type Associated with Reduced Vitamin D (Figs. 4.7 and 4.8)

Trichrome Vitiligo (Fig. 4.6)

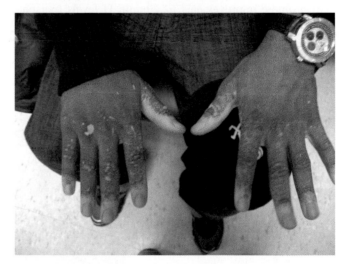

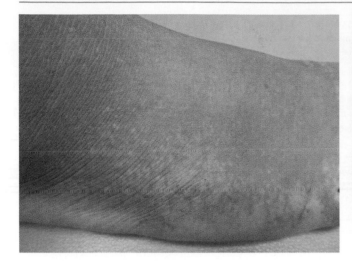

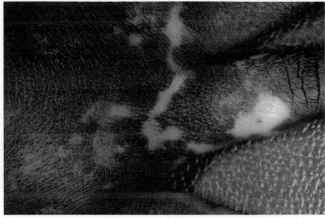

Many patients with vitiligo have very low 25 (OH) Vitamin D levels (<15 ng/dL), which may be linked to increased incidence of secondary autoimmunity, e.g., thyroid disease. In my practice I have noted that individuals of color with low vitamin D levels often manifest with clusters of pinpoint areas of depigmentation over the dorsal extremities, especially over the tops of the hands and as an extension in a speckled or diffuse pattern of lighter pigmentation from the plantar surface to the extensor foot (Figs. 4.7 and 4.8). Such patients do well with supplementation of vitamin D (orally and topically) and narrowband UVB therapy, which will promote improvements in vitamin D levels (personal observation) [9].

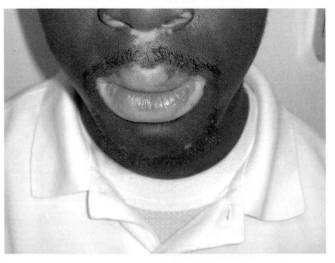

Prominence of Vitiligo in Individuals of Color (Figs. 4.9–4.11)

Vitiligo vulgaris can affect any site; however, in individuals of color, lesions are more visible (Figs. 4.9 and 4.10). One site where this is especially true is the lips (Fig. 4.11). Some authors estimate that half of children with vitiligo will have oral mucosal involvement, which may mark risk of disease progression [10]. Vitiliginous lips are rarely cosmetically noticeable in Caucasian and Asian children unless depigmentation extends to the perioral skin, but are very visible in Hispanic, Indian, and Black individuals, as noted in the Figs. 4.9–4.11. Standard vitiligo therapies such as topical corticosteroids or excimer laser can effect some repigmentation, but full repigmentation is rare in such cases (Table 4.3).

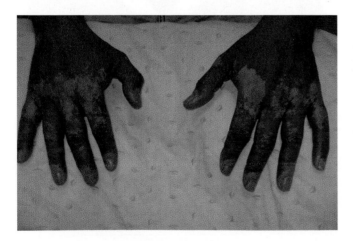

Table 4.3 Treatment paradigm for vitiligo in children

Localized lesions: Topical corticosteroids (high potency for 2 months twice-daily followed by strength reduction or pulsed usage); topical calcineurin inhibitors twice-daily or topical corticosteroid once daily and topical calcipotriene 0.005% once daily are alternative regimens; excimer laser for resistant lesions
Segmental lesions: Calcineurin inhibitors twice-daily (especially tacrolimus); High potency corticosteroids with or without calcipotriene 0.005% can be used alternatively; excimer laser is slower than for other types of vitiligo, but effective
Generalized vitiligo
Stabilize unstable cases using narrowband UVB (3 months) and care for any identified medical issues or deficiencies; oral corticosteroids to stabilize severe cases using monthly pulses for 2–5 days
Topical therapy can be used in limited cases or for specific lesions
Narrowband UVB twice weekly to thrice weekly or PUVA for repigmentation [22]
Excimer laser for residual areas of hypopigmentation

Follicular Repigmentation and Border Hyperpigmentation (Fig. 4.12)

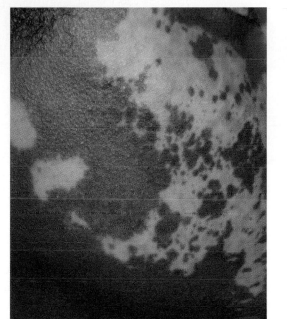

Repigmentation in vitiliginous lesions can occur through repigmentation from melanocytes in the dermis of the lesion, from melanocytes in the hair follicle or from migration of melanocytes from the border of the lesion resulting in fine-diffuse repigmentation, follicular repigmentation or hyperpigmentation of the vitiliginous border, the latter two types being demonstrated in Fig. 4.12. The speed of repigmentation is fastest with diffuse types and slowest from the border, however, follicular repigmentation and border repigmentation are the more likely to be sustained long term [11].

Erythema Dyschromicum Perstans (Figs. 4.13 and 4.14)

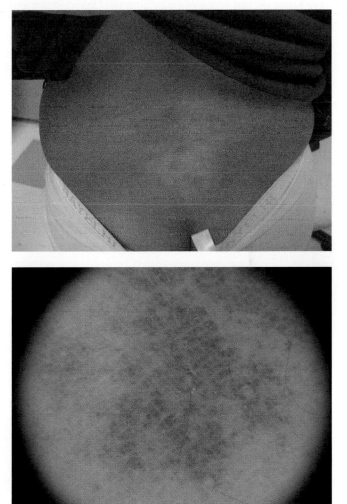

Erythema Dyschromicum Perstans, also known as ashy dermatosis or los senescientos, is a chronic inflammatory disorder of the skin that causes initially plaques with

Table 4.4 Work-up and treatment for erythema dyschromicum perstans

Physical examination (with dermoscopy demonstrating pigment dots in the dermis), with special care to identify ingested agents and medication triggers
Biopsy for H and E
Patch testing to identify possible causative contact allergens
Avoidance of any identified triggers, exacerbants and/or allergens
Sun protection
Topical medications: Dapsone 5% gel, Mid-potency corticosteroids (rarely effective)
Oral medications: Dapsone, Clofazamine, Hydroxychloroquine

erythematous borders that are soon replaced by gray-brown areas of hyperpigmentation. The disease occurs in all races, with increased prevalence in Hispanics. In Fig. 4.13, a Hispanic female teenager with biopsy proven Erythema Dyschromicum Perstans is depicted. Lesions in pre-pubertal children have a strong tendency towards spontaneous clearance based on two series of cases from the United States and Spain [12, 13]. However, when therapy is needed, a variety of agents, including clofazamine have been described to have variable success. Patch testing can identify inciting or aggravating agents, which should be withdrawn from the child's environment (Table 4.4).

Erythema Dyschromicum Perstans, histologically, is a deposition of pigment in the dermis with melanophages. Dermoscopy demonstrates packets of pigmentation in the dermis as noted in this dermoscopic photo of lesions from the same 16-year-old Hispanic girl shown in Fig. 4.14.

Progressive Macular Hypomelanosis (Fig. 4.15)

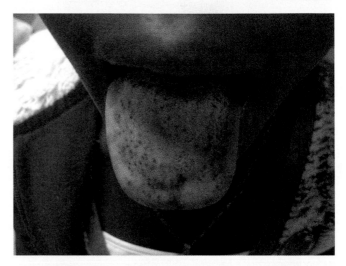

The Black adolescent in Fig. 4.15 demonstrates hypopigmentation on the back that is consistent with progressive macular hypomelanosis. Potassium hydroxide preparation is negative, excluding active tinea versicolor.

Progressive macular hypomelanosis has been recently described and is a disorder in which annular areas hypopig-

mentation occurs on the trunk over the V of the chest and back. Lesions are noted in teenagers and young adults of color, including Hispanic and Black children, in the United States. The etiology is unknown but may relate to overgrowth of *Proprionobacterium* species on the skin. Therapies including oral minocycline, topical clindamycin or benzoyl peroxide and narrowband ultraviolet B light for repigmentation (after other agents have been initiated) have been described [14, 15].

Oral Papillary Hyperpigmentation (Fig. 4.16)

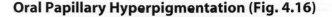

Oral papillary hyperpigmentation (Fig. 4.16) can be noted in normal children of color. Reports of benign pigmentation of the fungiform papillae include a well-circumscribed patch, few scattered lesions and pigmentation of all the fungiform papillae. Dermoscopy resembling rose petals has been reported [16]. This finding may be very common in individuals who are Black, but is rare in Caucasians and Asians. An association has been seen with hemochromatosis, iron deficiency, and scleroderma. The differential diagnosis would include oral acanthosis nigricans, melanoma, black hairy tongue, Peutz–Jegher syndrome, and Addison disease [17–19]. This can be distinguished from lingual fungiform papillae hypertrophy (Fig. 4.17) seen in viral syndromes and with high dose oral cyclosporine A for renal transplantation [20], which is generally not pigmented.

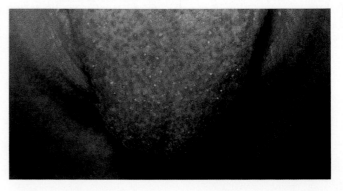

Frictional Hyperpigmentation (Fig. 4.18)

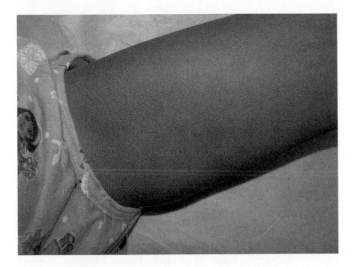

Frictional skin tone changes occur in children on the inner thighs (Fig. 4.18), lower buttock, and with breast development in the female underarm. Overweight children and children who experience frictional dermatitis are likely to see such changes. In Caucasians a yellow-tan color may be noted, while in African American children, as noted here, hyperpigmentation, follicular prominence, and lichenoid papules may be seen.

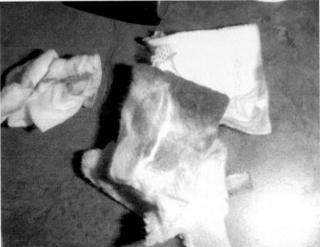

SCURF-Acquired Hyperpigmentation Due to Retention Hyperkeratosis and Terra Firma (Figs. 4.19–4.22)

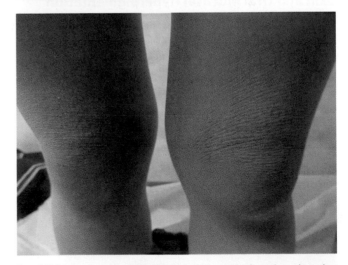

In children of color SCURF takes on a dark coloration that can mimic Confluent and Reticulated Hyperkeratosis (Fig. 4.19). Therefore, a trial of scrubbing with an alcohol pad in the office is needed in all children presenting with

Confluent and Reticulated Hyperkeratosis, to rule out dirt (Figs. 4.20 and 4.21). Mimicry of confluent and reticulated papillomatosis is common in SCURF of Black individuals, while acquired ichthyosis may be suspected in Caucasian children with SCURF (Fig. 4.22).

Forehead Callous—Prayer Induced (Fig. 4.23)

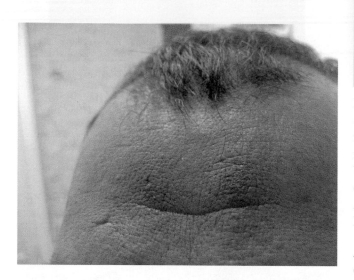

Devout Muslims pray with their forehead touching a prayer rug. This individual demonstrates a callosity or lichen simplex chronicus from prayer (Fig. 4.23). This is usually noted in individuals of Arab or South Indian background.

Skin and Oral Mucosal Hyperpigmentation (Figs. 4.24 and 4.25)

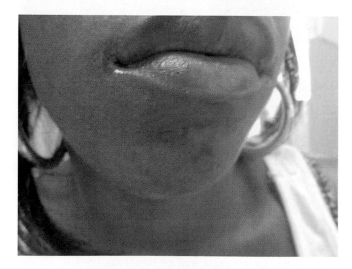

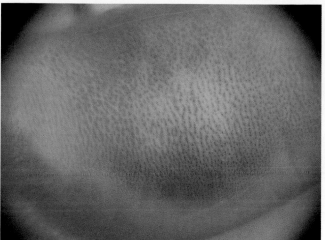

Pigmentary alterations are often noted after insult, trauma, and/or inflammation of the skin in individuals of color. This is noted on the skin as seen with picking of acne and plucking unwanted chin hairs as noted in Fig. 4.24 flares, but can be seen in the oral mucosa as noted in the dermoscopic photo of an orolabial melanotic macule on the oral mucosa in an African American girl who habitually bites and sucks her lower lip (Fig. 4.25).

Cupping (Fig. 4.26)

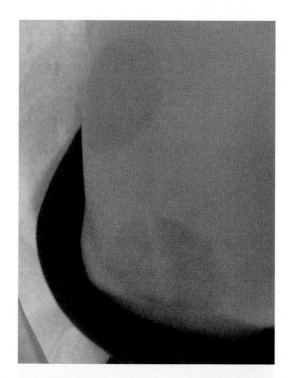

Chinese traditional therapies use heated glass cups which create purpura at the base through suction (Fig. 4.26). Similar cupping therapies have been used in a variety of cultures. In Yiddish cupping is termed bankis.

Acquired Ochronosis (Fig. 4.27)

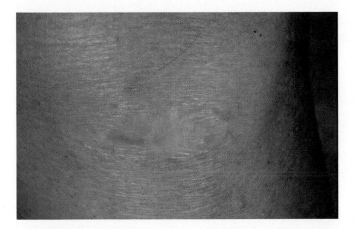

Acquired ochronosis (Fig. 4.27) can occur when hydroquinones of 4% strength or higher are used on a prolonged basis. A blue tinge will be noted overlying hydroquinone-induced hypopigmentation. As melasma is more common in women of color, ochronosis from hydroquinone usage seems to occur in this grouping as well, although reporting in teenage years is uncommon.

References

1. Leung AK, Robson WL, Liu EK, Kao CP, Fong JH, Leong AG, Cheung BC, Wong AH, Chen SY (2007) Melanonychia striata in Chinese children and adults. Int J Dermatol 46:920–922
2. Hashimoto K (1971) Ultrastructure of the human toenail: I. Proximal nail matrix. J Invest Dermatol 56:235–246
3. Sachdeva S, Sachdeva S, Kapoor P (2011) Laugier-Hunziker syndrome: a rare cause of oral and acral pigmentation. J Cutan Aesthet Surg 4:58–60
4. Tosti A, Daniel RC III, Piraccini BM, Iorizzo M (2010) Color atlas of nails. Springer, New York, p 98
5. Shah S, Alexis A, Silverberg NB (2007) Treatment of vitiligo in children of color. Asian Pigment Bull 2:4–17
6. Silverberg NB (2010) Update on childhood vitiligo. Curr Opin Pediatr 22:445–452
7. Ducharme EE, Silverberg NB (2008) Selected applications of technology in the pediatric dermatology office. Semin Cutan Med Surg 27:94–100
8. Hann SK, Kim YS, Yoo JH, Chun YS (2000) Clinical and histopathologic characteristics of trichrome vitiligo. J Am Acad Dermatol 42:589–596
9. Silverberg JI, Silverberg AI, Malka E, Silverberg NB (2010) A pilot study assessing the role of 25 hydroxy vitamin D levels in patients with vitiligo vulgaris. J Am Acad Dermatol 62:937–941
10. Ruiz-Maldonado R (2007) Hypomelanotic conditions of the newborn and infant. Dermatol Clin 25:373–382; ix
11. Parsad D, Pandhi R, Dogra S, Kumar B (2004) Clinical study of repigmentation patterns with different treatment modalities and their correlation with speed and stability of repigmentation in 352 vitiliginous patches. J Am Acad Dermatol 50:63–67
12. Silverberg NB, Herz J, Wagner A, Paller AS (2003) Erythema dyschromicum perstans in prepubertal children. Pediatr Dermatol 20:398–403
13. Torrelo A, Zaballos P, Colmenero I, Mediero IG, de Prada I, Zambrano A (2005) Erythema dyschromicum perstans in children: a report of 14 cases. J Eur Acad Dermatol Venereol 19:422–426
14. Wu XG, Xu AE, Luo XY, Song XZ (2010) A case of progressive macular hypomelanosis successfully treated with benzoyl peroxide plus narrow-band UVB. J Dermatolog Treat 21:367–368
15. Relyveld GN, Westerhof W, Woudenberg J, Kingswijk M, Langenberg M, Vandenbroucke-Grauls CM, Bos JD, Savelkoul PH (2010) Progressive macular hypomelanosis is associated with a putative Propionibacterium species. J Invest Dermatol 130:1182–1184
16. Mukamal LV, Ormiga P, Ramos-E-Silva M (2012) Dermoscopy of the pigmented fungiform papillae of the tongue. J Dermatol 39(4):397–399
17. Rangwala S, Doherty CB, Katta R (2010) Laugier-Hunziker syndrome: a case report and review of the literature. Dermatol Online J 16:9
18. Romiti R, Molina De Medeiros L (2010) Pigmented fungiform papillae of the tongue. Pediatr Dermatol 27(4):398–399
19. Pehoushek JF, Norton SA, Bliss RW (1999) Black taste buds. Arch Dermatol 135(594–595):597–598
20. Silverberg NB, Singh A, Echt AF, Laude TA (1996) Lingual fungiform papillae hypertrophy with cyclosporin A. Lancet 348(9032):967
21. Buka R, Friedman KA, Phelps RG, Silver L, Calero F, Rudikoff D (2001) Childhood longitudinal melanonychia: case reports and review of the literature. Mt Sinai J Med 68:331–335
22. Tlougan BE, Gonzalez ME, Mandal RV, Kundu RV, Skopicki D (2010) Erythema dyschromicum perstans. Dermatol Online J 16:17

Cutis Marmorata Telangiectatica Congenita (Figs. 5.1–5.3)

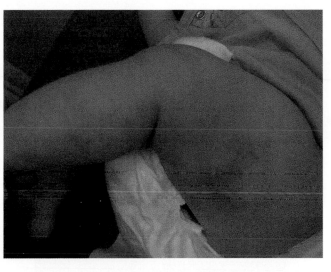

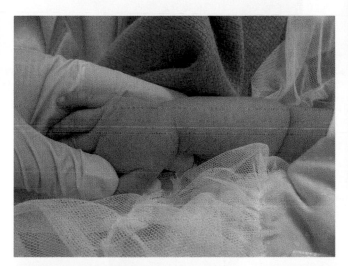

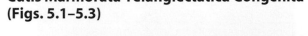

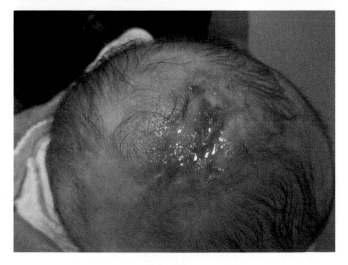

Cutis marmorata telangiectatica congenital (CMTC) is a vascular malformation that can cover part or all of the body with a reticulate prominent vasculature (Figs. 5.1–5.3), which mimics livedo reticularis. Diagnostic criteria include, major criteria: (1) Congenital reticulated (marmorated) erythema, (2) Absence of venectasia, (3) Unresponsiveness to local warming and minor criteria: (a) fading of erythema within 2 years, (b) telangiectasia, (c) port wine stain in an area unaffected, (d) ulceration, and (e) atrophy [1].

Lesions are often prominent over the legs and trunk and an appearance of atrophy near vessels is not uncommon. Spontaneous improvement with age does occur through childhood and adolescence. As with other vascular malformations, it may be associated with limb asymmetry and structural defects. A prominent vascular pattern is associated with the appearance of atrophy, which is often an optical illusion associated with the vascular ectasia, and may be more prominent in darker skin tones.

N.B. Silverberg, *Atlas of Pediatric Cutaneous Biodiversity: Comparative Dermatologic Atlas of Pediatric Skin of All Colors*, DOI 10.1007/978-1-4614-3564-8_5, © Springer Science+Business Media, LLC 2012

The Asian child in Figs. 5.1 and 5.2 with CMTC also has cutis aplasia and a congenital heart defect. Notably, the scalp hair obscures some of the CMTC pattern. This grouping of CMTC and cutis aplasia falls under the Adams–Oliver syndrome. Other types of anomalies associated with CMTC include limb asymmetry, Circle of Willis defects and Arnold Chiari malformations, macrocephaly, neurological changes, and syndactyly [1]. In this patient, the aplasia closed by secondary intention without grafting.

In the Hispanic child in Fig. 5.3, CMTC has a deep violaceous appearance, but skin pigmentation blunts the appearance of atrophy noted in lighter patients. CMTC cases appear uncommon in Black children.

Nevus Simplex (Fig. 5.4)

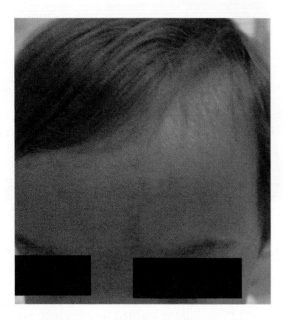

Nevus simplex (Fig. 5.4) is a very common vascular ectasia over the glabella, eyelids, and nuchal region, also termed "salmon patch," "angel kisses," "stork bites," and medial telangiectatica nevus. Blanching erythematous macules are noted in typical locations with localization can also be noted over the back, lower extremities, and lower lip. Lesions generally resolve on the face by 1 year of age. Nuchal lesions persist in most individuals, but are covered by hair as the child ages. Nevus simplex is most frequently noted in Caucasian children (non-Hispanic) (70.3%), but has been reported in children of color as well (Black 59.2% and Latin 67.9%) [2]. Glabellar lesions that are deep in coloration may not resolve and have been referred to as the medial fronto-facial capillary malformations [3]. Clearance with pulsed dye laser for nonresolving lesions is possible in all skin types; however, dyspigmentation is more likely in darker

individuals [4]. An association of extensive lesions with syndromes such as Beckwith-Wiedemann, macrocephaly-capillary malformation, odontodysplasia, and Roberts-SC phocomelia syndromes can be rarely noted.

Port Wine Stain (Figs. 5.5–5.8)

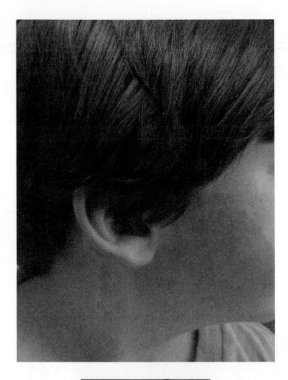

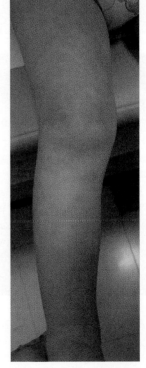

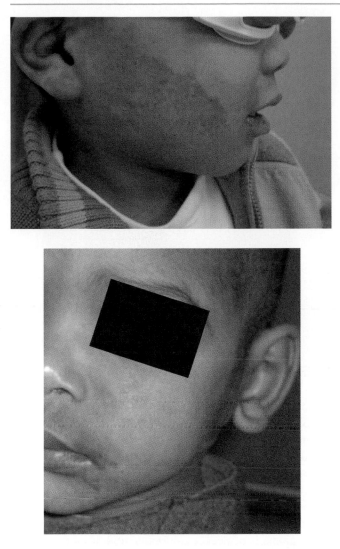

taking on the appearance of a light red wine. Because therapeutic response is better in the macular lesions of childhood, rather than in the thickened lesions of older patients, pulsed dye laser should be initiated early on [8].

Port wine stains that are segmental on the limbs as the one in Fig. 5.7 are more likely associated with limb defects such as lymphatic malformations and overgrowth. This Hispanic child with a port wine stain demonstrates that background pigmentation overlying tends to make the stain less bright red, favoring burgundy.

In the African American patient with a port wine stain (Fig. 5.8), pigment obscures the erythema extensively. In addition, the pigment acts as a partial filter to pulsed dye laser.

Port wine stains in individuals of all colors can respond to pulsed-dye laser therapy. However, in skin types IV and V (especially Indian patients), temporary postinflammatory hyperpigmentation (less likely hypopigmentation) can be noted after pulsed-dye laser therapy. Type V and VI skin in African American patients can blister, resulting in textural alterations [9]. This complication has been reduced by cryogen spray devices and other forms of dynamic cooling, however, test spots are often ideal prior to treating large lesions in dark individuals.

As with all postinflammatory changes, strict sun protection and judicious usage of hydroquinone agents or other lightening products may minimize discolorations [10]. Sturge Weber syndrome seems to be rarely reported in Black children; however, gingival hypertrophy may be seen in such rare cases, exacerbated by phenytoin usage [11]. When lesions are not amenable to laser therapy, or laser therapy is not desired, cosmetic cover-up can be used.

Infantile Hemangiomas (Figs. 5.9–5.13)

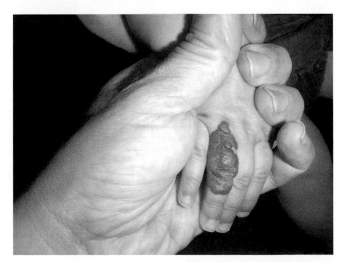

A port wine stain is a capillary vascular malformation that can occur focally, blotchy/segmentally, geographically or in a broad, generalized pattern. Associated glaucoma with V2 involvement, less so V1 facial segments, Sturge Weber syndrome with V1 facial segment [5], and limb hypertrophy/ lymphatic malformations (Klippel Trenauney syndrome) can be noted in association with port wine stains, the latter being associated with geographic lesions [6]. In the Caucasian patient with a port wine stain (Fig. 5.5), the true color that mimics port wine is noted. Lighter lesions are often more amenable to pulsed dye laser, however, even the deep port wine stains can respond to extensive pulsed-dye laser sessions. Response to pulsed dye laser is best in the V3 distribution [5]. Even years after therapy, individuals retain both lightening and less worry regarding their physical appearance, resulting in less psychological morbidity [7].

In the Asian patient the port wine stain (Fig. 5.6) is similar to that of the Caucasian, but is rarely as bright magenta,

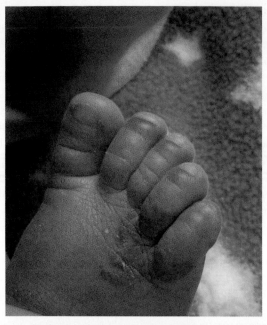

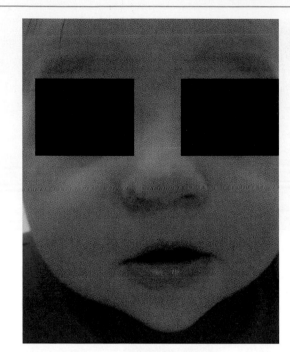

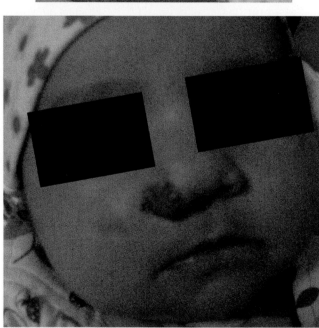

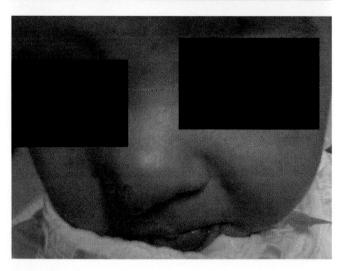

Infantile Hemangiomas are benign vascular tumors that grow from 2 to 9 months of age, the majority of enlargement being complete in the first 3 months of activity (Figs. 5.9 and 5.10), and begin to involute during the second year of life. Involution is complete in 50% by 5 years of age. Superficial (Fig. 5.9) and deeper variants (Fig. 5.11) exist and compound lesions (superficial and deep) may be seen. In the Caucasian female infant in Fig. 5.9, it is easily noted that the vascular tumor is bright red. Deeper lesions take on a blue tinge. In the African American infant in Fig. 5.10, one can appreciate that the hemangioma is of deeper coloration, almost mimicking the depth of color of a port wine stain (Fig. 5.10).

Fair skin (white, non-Hispanic) and female sex are associated with hemangiomas of infancy, as are prematurity, placenta previa, multiple gestations, advanced maternal age, and pre-eclampsia [12].

The lesion over the nasal bridge in the Hispanic infant in Fig. 5.11 grew rapidly from age 2 to 3 months, distorting the nasal structure (Fig. 5.12). Untreated such lesions can cause Cyranno deformities, ulceration, and scarring. This lesion shrank rapidly on oral Propranolol (Figs. 5.13 and 5.14) as noted in this photo 2 and 4 months after induction, allowing preservation of the nasal shape. Hemangiomas of infancy in Hispanic children are more likely to require medical attention, because they are more likely to present with segmental lesions, complex lesions involving the mucous membranes and to have a greater morbidity, including the presence of associated anomalies such as PHACE syndrome than any other segment of the population. Complications were noted in 47% of Hispanic hemangiomas of infancy. Forty percent of PHACE cases and 50% of the spinal involvement case were Hispanic, although Hispanic hemangiomas only constituted 74 of the 472 lesions (15.6%) in the case series.

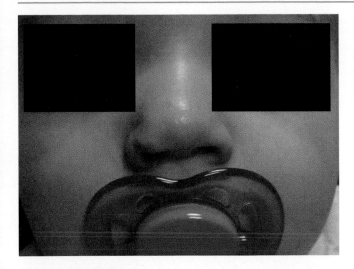

Infantile hemangiomas are less likely to be noted in Black children, being present at birth in 0.1% of Black vs. 0.7% of Caucasian children [2]. Underrepresentation in number of cases is also accompanied by a lower likelihood to receive systemic therapy in Blacks (24.1%) vs. Hispanic (32.3%) and white non-Hispanic patients (31.1%) [12].

Sequelae of Hemangiomas of Infancy (Fig. 5.15)

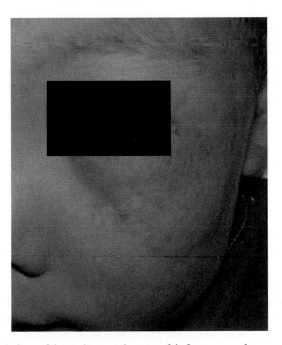

Resolution of large hemangiomas of infancy may be complicated by scarring. In this Asian child who presented at 2 years of age, textural surface changes including atrophy, dyspigmentation, and loss of skin turgor and wrinkling can be noted (Fig. 5.15). A recent study of Chinese children with hemangiomas of infancy showed that facial hemangiomas in Asian

children were 2.66 times as likely as other sites to have complications. For each 10 cm² increase in size, there was a 9% increased risk of complications and a 28% increased risk of need for corticosteroid therapy [13]. This child demonstrates a segmental hemangioma, which placed him at increased risk of complications such as PHACES syndrome (posterior fossa brain malformations, hemangioma of infancy, arterial anomalies, coarctation of the aorta and cardiac defects, and eye abnormalities). The following risk factors were identified for hemangiomas in the Chinese population: lower levels of maternal education, mother engaged in manual labor, multiple gestations, maternal periconceptional medication usage, e.g., progesterone, clomifid, and a positive family history of hemangiomas [13].

Infantile Hemangioma: Late Therapy with Propranolol (Figs. 5.16 and 5.17)

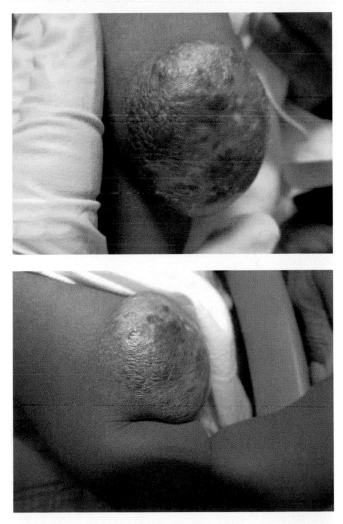

In this African American child who presented at 13 months with a deep infantile hemangioma, one can note that dyspigmentation can occur in overlying lesions (Fig. 5.16), especially in children of color, exacerbated by prior ulceration. After 1 month Propranolol orally, the lesion is less erythematous and has become exceedingly soft (Fig. 5.17). Abnormal surface texture and coloration from old ulceration are retained despite the rapid onset of involution. Earlier institution of therapy produces more optimal cosmesis.

Rapidly Involuting Congenital Hemangioma (Fig. 5.18)

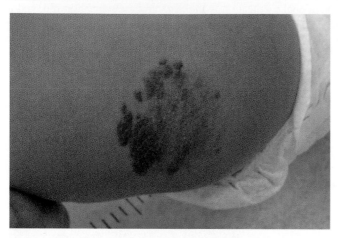

Hemangiomas of infancy that occur in utero or early on, but begin to resolve in early infancy are termed rapidly involuting congenital hemangiomas (Fig. 5.18). These lesions look clinically similar to hemangiomas of infancy but negative for the immunohistochemical marker, GLUT1 (glucose transporter type 1). It is notable that this hemangioma is deeper in coloration than those seen in Caucasian children. Rapid deflation of lesions often results in redundant skin and scar formation.

Spider Angioma (Figs. 5.19 and 5.20)

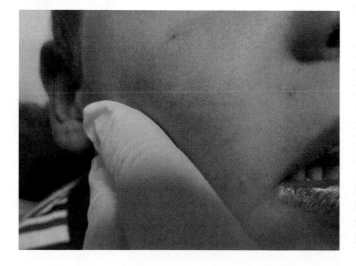

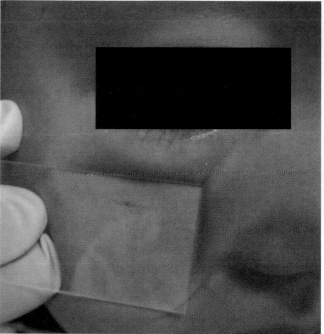

Spider angiomas are common and usually self-healing vascular ectasias over the central face and dorsal hands in lighter-skinned (Caucasian) children and adolescents (Fig. 5.19). Adults and infants are rarely affected, suggesting that these are induced by environmental traumas (e.g., ultraviolet light) and they resolve with age. Relationship to cirrhosis is not noted in children [14]. Here we can see blanching of the lesion with diascopy (Fig. 5.20), which aids in diagnosis. These lesions are not noted in children of Fitzpatrick phototypes IV–VI, probably due to intrinsic photoprotection. Pulsed dye laser can induce more rapid clearance.

The nevus anemicus is a vascular malformation in which vessels constrict, probably due to abnormal autonomic stimulation. Diascopy with a slide will even these areas out with the surrounding skin, similar to the effect seen in spider angiomas. The anemic effect can also be noted around developing hemangiomas of infancy. The anemic effect is rare in children of color as is the nevus anemicus [15].

Another form of vascular malformation noted in a specific group of color is the cerebral cavernous malformation syndrome which is familial in one-third of cases. Lesions have been described in type 1 in Southwestern (Northern New Mexico) Hispanic-Americans of Mexican descent due to a founder effect in the gene from Spanish settlers (Q455X mutation of CCM1). The disease has a high penetrance and lesions can be found on gradient echo magnetic resonance imaging [16]. Cerebral cavernous malformations are low-flow lesions which are well-circumscribed sinusoidal spaces lined by a single layer endothelium and separated by a collagenous matrix without smooth muscle. No cutaneous features are noted. Neurological features include seizures, headaches, hemorrhage, or focal neurologic deficits [17].

References

1. Kienast AK, Hoeger PH (2009) Cutis marmorata telangiectatica congenita: a prospective study of 27 cases and review of the literature with proposal of diagnostic criteria. Clin Exp Dermatol 34:319–323

2. Alper JC, Holmes LB (1983) The incidence and significance of birthmarks in a cohort of 4,641 newborns. Pediatr Dermatol 1(1):58–68

3. Sillard L, Léauté-Labreze C, Mazereeuw-Hautier J, Viseux V, Barbarot S, Vabres P, Bessis D, Martin L, Lorette G, Berthier F, Lacour JP (2011) Medial fronto-facial capillary malformations. J Pediatr 158(5):836–841

4. Garrett AB, Shieh S (2000) Treatment of vascular lesions in pigmented skin with the pulsed dye laser. J Cutan Med Surg 4:36–39

5. Hennedige AA, Quaba AA, Al-Nakib K (2008) Sturge-Weber syndrome and dermatomal facial port-wine stains: incidence, association with glaucoma, and pulsed tunable dye laser treatment effectiveness. Plast Reconstr Surg 121:1173–1180

6. Maari C, Frieden IJ (2004) Klippel-Trénaunay syndrome: the importance of "geographic stains" in identifying lymphatic disease and risk of complications. J Am Acad Dermatol 51:391–398

7. Hansen K, Kreiter CD, Rosenbaum M, Whitaker DC, Arpey CJ (2003) Long-term psychological impact and perceived efficacy of pulsed-dye laser therapy for patients with port-wine stains. Dermatol Surg 29:49–55

8. Goh CL (2000) Flashlamp-pumped pulsed dye laser (585 nm) for the treatment of portwine stains—a study of treatment outcome in 94 Asian patients in Singapore. Singapore Med J 41:24–28

9. Ashinoff R, Geronemus RG (1992) Treatment of a port-wine stain in a black patient with the pulsed dye laser. J Dermatol Surg Oncol 18:147–148

10. Sharma VK, Khandpur S (2007) Efficacy of pulsed dye laser in facial port-wine stains in Indian patients. Dermatol Surg 33:560–566

11. Perkins TM, Duncan WK, Hill WJ, Krolls SO (1992) The Sturge-Weber syndrome: a case involving a 13-year-old black male. Ann Dent 51:40–43

12. Hemangioma Investigator Group, Haggstrom AN, Drolet BA, Baselga E, Chamlin SL, Garzon MC, Horii KA, Lucky AW, Mancini AJ, Metry DW, Newell B, Nopper AJ, Frieden IJ (2007) Prospective study of infantile hemangiomas: demographic, prenatal, and perinatal characteristics. J Pediatr 150:291–294

13. Li J, Chen X, Zhao S, Hu X, Chen C, Ouyang F, Liu Q, Ding R, Shi Q, Su J, Kuang Y, Chang J, Li F, Xie H (2011) Demographic and clinical characterisatics and risk factors for infantile hemangioma: a Chinese case-control study. Arch Dermatol 147:1049–1056

14. Alderson MR (1963) Spider naevi—their incidence in healthy school children. Arch Dis Child 38:286–288

15. Davies MG, Greaves MW, Coutts A, Black AK (1981) Nevus oligemicus. A variant of nevus anemicus. Arch Dermatol 117:111–113

16. Mindea SA, Yang BP, Shenkar R, Bendok B, Batjer HH, Awad IA (2006) Cerebral cavernous malformations: clinical insights from genetic studies. Neurosurg Focus 21:e1

17. Petersen TA, Morrison LA, Schrader RM, Hart BL (2010) Familial versus sporadic cavernous malformations: differences in developmental venous anomaly association and lesion phenotype. AJNR Am J Neuroradiol 31:377–382

Psoriasis (Figs. 6.1–6.14)

Psoriasis vulgaris is the prototypical papulosquamous disorder. Three types affect children—infantile psoriasis, psoriasis with early onset, and psoriatic arthritis. One third of psoriatic cases begin in childhood, with an average onset in grade school. One third of cases are precipitated by an upper respiratory infection, often *Streptococcal* [1]. In a Southern California cohort of children from 2007 to 2008, point prevalence of psoriasis was 29 non-Hispanic whites, 20 Asian/Pacific Islanders, 16 Hispanic whites, and 6 blacks per 10,000 patients [2]. Caucasian psoriatic children may have a slightly earlier onset than other groupings, possibly due to stronger genetic burden, and more family history of disease [3]. However, psoriasis is associated with higher body mass index [4] and the epidemic of obesity strongly affects children of color; thus, there may be a trend in the future to rising incidence of psoriasis in children of color, as well as Caucasian children.

In my practice, a majority of the most severely affected teenagers already manifest obesity and metabolic syndrome (see Chap. 15). Screening for hyperlipidemia in severe childhood psoriasis is needed. Referral to weight down programs may be helpful to reduce cardiovascular risk factors in psoriatic children and teenagers.

Pityriasis Amiantacea (Fig. 6.1)

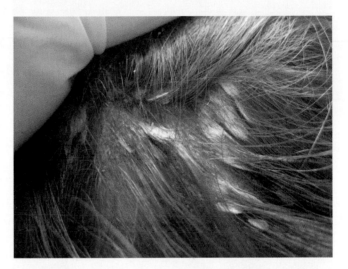

Pityriasis amiantacea (Fig. 6.1) is a papulosquamous scalp disorder in which thick hyperkeratosis becomes attached to hair shafts, creating a caked on appearance similar to inflammatory forms of tinea capitis. Children are primarily affected, especially Caucasian and Arabic children [5]. Hispanic children may be less affected and it is exceedingly rare in African American children. Salicylic acid and oil-based products are used to soften scales, thereby freeing them of scales from the hairs, allowing clearance of the scalp and unmasking of scalp disease, without accidental removal of hair. Like all forms of scalp hyperkeratosis, fungal culture and/or potassium hydroxide preparation are needed in childhood to identify tinea capitis mimicking the dermatosis. In Scandinavian children with Pityriasis amiantacea, psoriasis vulgaris is statistically more likely to occur than in the general population [6].

N.B. Silverberg, *Atlas of Pediatric Cutaneous Biodiversity: Comparative Dermatologic Atlas of Pediatric Skin of All Colors*, DOI 10.1007/978-1-4614-3564-8_6, © Springer Science+Business Media, LLC 2012

Facial Psoriasis (Figs. 6.2 and 6.3)

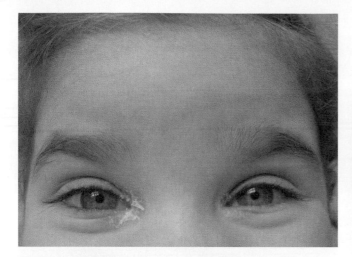

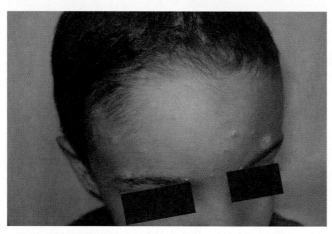

Forehead Psoriasis and Postinflammatory Hyperpigmentation (Figs. 6.4 and 6.5)

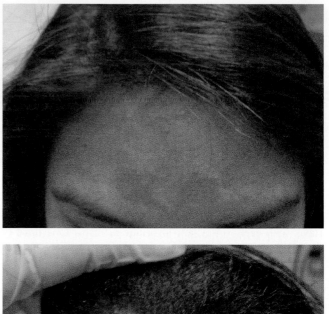

While most psoriasis in childhood is plaque type, localization of plaques is common on the face in childhood (38%) (Figs. 6.2 and 6.3), including the periocular areas [7]. This results in a greater psychosocial morbidity for young children with the disease. Facial psoriasis is no more noticeable in darker children than lighter children, but the residual hyperpigmentation after lesional clearance is worse in children of color. Mid-potency topical corticosteroids with or without calcipotriene as well as topical calcineurin inhibitors are very helpful in clearance of such lesions, but limitations in periocular lesional therapy include inability to apply high-potency corticosteroid products due to risk of skin atrophy and glaucoma, irritation from rubbing products into the eye, and poor penetration of agents through micaceous scale.

Psoriasis is likely to affect Black children similarly to Caucasian and Hispanic children in lesional type and distribution [8]. However, the incidence of psoriasis is far lower in Black children, a trend that persists into adulthood (2); the adult black population (1.3%) is only about half of that of the adult Caucasian non-Hispanic populus (2.5%) [9].

In Caucasian children, postinflammatory erythema is common and in Asian and African American children, lesional and postinflammatory hyperpigmentation. Postinflammatory pigmentary alteration is nearly universal but more prominent in Asian children and children of color with psoriasis of childhood, driving emotional distress [7].

Psoriatic lesions in all age groups affect the scalp as the number one site, and isolated scalp disease is the third most common type of pediatric psoriasis after plaque and infantile types. On the scalp, the presence of psoriatic lesions can mimic tinea capitis. One of the clues to the diagnosis of psoriasis is the presence of lesions of the anterior scalp extending forward onto the hairline and forehead (Figs. 6.4 and 6.5). In the African American teenager in Fig. 6.5 we can see scalp hyperkeratosis similar to Caucasian patients, with extension of lesions onto the forehead. Lesions are darker and more violaceous than those noted in Caucasian individuals. Such lesions often leave behind extensive postinflammatory hypopigmentary alterations in individuals of Fitzpatrick types 3–5 and erythema in children of color. When hypopigmentation is Wood's lamp enhancing, one should consider inflammatory vitiligo as an alternative diagnosis. Ultraviolet light (e.g., narrowband UVB) can aid in lesional clearance and promote repigmentation. Rapid introduction of effective therapies can help minimize postinflammatory changes and psychological morbidity. Baseline quality of life may be poorest in Hispanic individuals with psoriasis, although childhood data is lacking [10].

Scale in Psoriasis (Figs. 6.6–6.9)

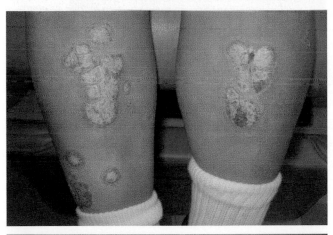

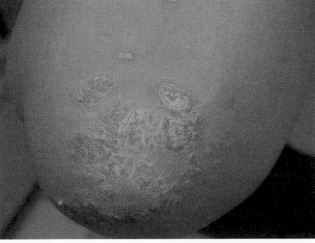

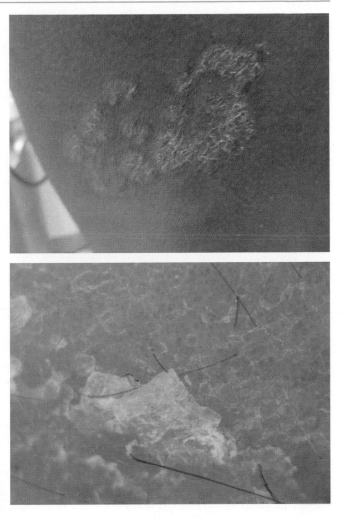

Micaceous scale is the term for the white, thick flaky scales noted primarily in older children, especially Caucasians (Fig. 6.6). This type of scale is associated with plaque-type psoriasis, in which lesions especially affect the elbows and knees. Micaceous Scale is not often noted in very young children (Fig. 6.7) and Black patients (Fig. 6.8). With dermoscopy, the Auspitz sign can be observed, i.e., pinpoint vessels underneath micaceous scale (Fig. 6.9). In this way, one does not need to scrape off the scale to observe the pinpoint bleeding. Removal of scale via keratolytic agents is required in order to treat the inflamed base of the lesion.

Guttate Psoriasis (Fig. 6.10)

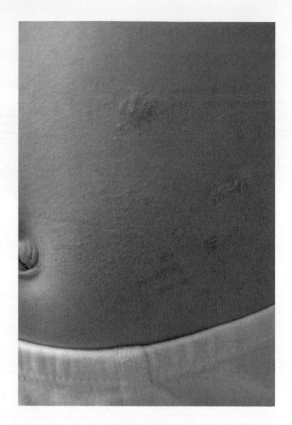

Psoriasis and Postinflammatory Hypopigmentation (Fig. 6.11)

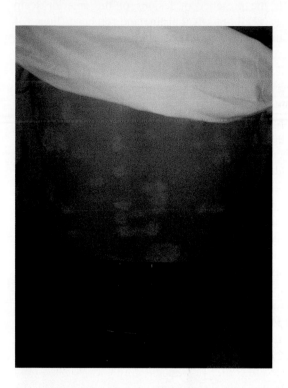

Guttate psoriasis accounts for one third of cases in younger patients. Guttate lesions are often small, red in Caucasian children (Fig. 6.10) to violaceous in Black children. Guttate lesions are usually numerous and clustered over the torso. Therapy is difficult for these cases, as the number of lesions makes topical therapy cumbersome. Oral antibiotics (e.g., erythromycin, azithromycin) may aid in this type of psoriasis, as guttate flares can be precipitated by group A beta hemolytic streptococcal infections.

When phototherapy or coal tar is used in pediatric psoriasis of Caucasians and Hispanic/Latino children, a light halo may begin to form (Fig. 6.11). In children, most of these halos are hypopigmentation, but the form described in adults has been a vasospastic phenomenon, i.e., Woronoff rings, in some cases. One hypothesis for Woronoff rings is diffusion of prostaglandin synthesis inhibitors related to phototherapy. In childhood, it is my observation that light rings around psoriasis form either as postinflammatory changes are unmasked by lesion clearance and postinflammatory hypopigmentation or by lack of tanning by active lesions.

Psoriasis of the Nail (Fig. 6.12)

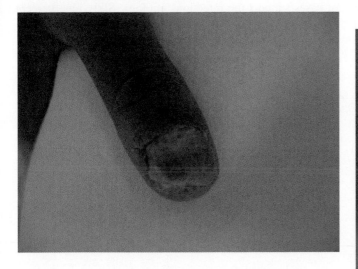

Inverse Psoriasis/Nappy Psoriasis (Figs. 6.13 and 6.14)

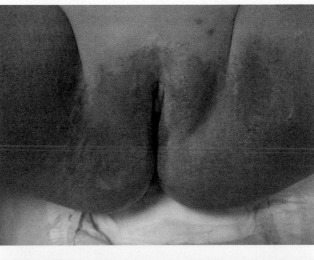

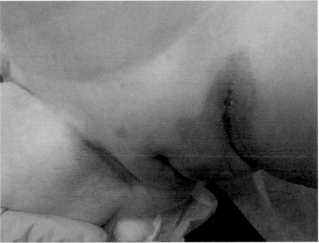

Psoriasis of the nail unit is a cosmetically disfiguring form that is present in 76.9% of Caucasian adult psoriatics and 85.7% of psoriatics with joint involvement [11]. Lower incidence of nail psoriasis is reported in childhood including 25.5% of Chinese children with psoriasis under the age of 14 years [12] to 37.81% of Kuwaiti children with psoriasis [13]. Typical clinical appearance includes nail pitting (61.84%), onycholysis (30.26%), subungual hyperkeratosis (13.16%) that is fungal culture and PAS stain negative (although superimposed onychomycosis can occur in the setting of psoriasis), crumbling, and discoloration (7.9%) such as oil spots under the nail. Subungual hyperkeratosis and oil spotting are demonstrated in Fig. 6.12 of a finger in an African American boy. Pigmented skin does not seem to obscure the clinical features of nail psoriasis.

In the differential diagnosis of nail psoriasis is trachyonychia, the 20 nail dystrophy is a form of nail pitting which progresses to thinning and dystrophy of the nails, and is associated with alopecia areata and psoriasis. Nail pitting is seen in 10.5% of children with alopecia areata, but the pitting is rarely associated with the dystrophic changes of trachyonychia [14]. While psoriasis is often triggered in a nail unit by trauma, trachyonychia indiscriminately affects all or most of the nails. Trachyonychia has been thought to be a form of nail psoriasis; however, the natural history is toward resolution spontaneously at 6 years in at least half of children. Therefore, trachyonychia seems to be more likely a form of alopecia areata-like inflammation of the nail unit [15]. Although the cases reported in the literature are primarily Caucasian and Asian children, in New York City most of the cases I see are in children who are Hispanic or African American, with similarly excellent spontaneous resolution by 6 years time, regardless of therapy.

Lesion appearance of psoriasis in the axillae, groin, and intergluteal cleft are termed inverse psoriasis (Figs. 6.13 and 6.14). This variant, which is common in infancy ("nappy" or napkin psoriasis), is often lacking in typical scale due to moisture in the intertriginous areas and is often more violaceous than other sites. Anecdotally, infantile psoriasis is mostly noted in Caucasian infants in my practice and rare in Black infants, but I can find no reference reviewing racial differences in incidence for this type.

Differentiation from other forms of diaper dermatitis can be made based on thick violaceous plaques (more erythematous than seborrheic dermatitis) that are well demarcated and involve the genitalia, intertriginous folds, and inner thighs continuously and evenly. Maceration and deep erythema can be due to *Candida albicans* overgrowth on lesion skin. In teenagers, hyperhidrosis can be an exacerbating factor. I have observed that some of these cases will culture bacteria from the throat and/or rectal region, thus bacterial culture or empirical trial of oral antibiotics may aid in clearance.

Infantile cases often resolve with time, but inverse psoriasis in older children does not spontaneously clear in most cases. Usage of topical anti-inflammatory agents (especially low to mid-potency corticosteroids, topical calcipotriene, or topical calcineurin inhibitors) can be paired with topical antifungals is a standard therapeutic regimen for these regions. Avoidance of high-potency products in these regions helps prevent striae formation [16].

Pityriasis Rosea (Figs. 6.15 and 6.16)

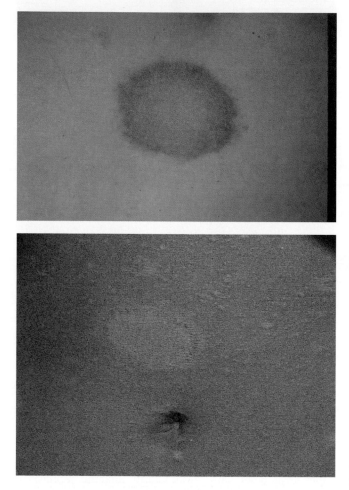

Pityriasis Rosea is a common papulosquamous reaction pattern of childhood. Lesions begin with one larger plaque called the herald patch (which is a misnomer, since it is raised with pityriasiform scale at the border), and progress over a 6-week time period. Lesions are papules and plaques occurring along the lines of cleavage on the chest, back, and abdomen and proximal extremities. Lesions follow a so-called "Christmas tree" pattern over the back, while wrapping around the inner arm like bands. Resolution over a 6–8-week time period is usual.

Linkage to upper respiratory infections (33%) such as HHV-6 and HHV-7 has been suggested; however, the data is equivocal. Seasonal peaks in Spring and Fall and clustering of cases support the infectious etiology. Sixty-nine percent of children will have pruritus, often requiring symptomatic therapy with oral antihistamines and/or topical corticosteroids. The first photo (Fig. 6.15) demonstrates the typical salmon-colored plaques of Caucasian pityriasis rosea. In childhood, while 67% of cases have centrally located lesions on the trunk, the other third of cases have diffuse, peripheral, or inverse lesion localization. Inverse cases may have a more prolonged course than other subtypes [17].

The second photograph demonstrates the herald patch, seen in half of childhood cases [17] and the localization of lesions within cleavage lines. As can be noted, this Hispanic teenager does not have salmon-colored lesions, but rather lesions that are erythematous to flesh-colored (Fig. 6.16). The pityriasiform scale is easily noted in these lesions.

"Atypical" Pityriasis Rosea (Figs. 6.17 and 6.18)

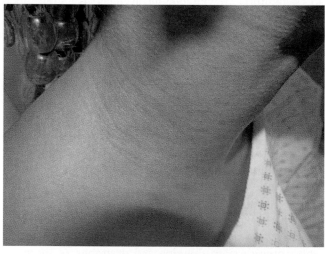

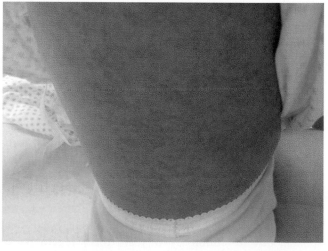

In the African American children in Figs. 6.17 and 6.18 one can note atypical site of lesions extending onto the neck and lower face. Lesions in African American children often involve the face (30%) and the scalp (8%). Many children of color have papular lesions, mimicking a viral exanthem. Postinflammatory pigmentary alteration (48% hyperpigmentation and 29% hypopigmentation) is very common in Black children and often lasts far longer than the original disease [18]. It is unclear whether usage of topical corticosteroids and antihistamines for lesion therapy reduces the risk of pigmentary alteration. However, these agents do provide symptomatic improvement in pruritic individuals. In all sexually active individuals, especially those with unusual presentations of pityriasis rosea such as distal extremity lesions, testing for secondary syphilis is recommended.

Unilateral Laterothoracic Exanthem (Fig. 6.19)

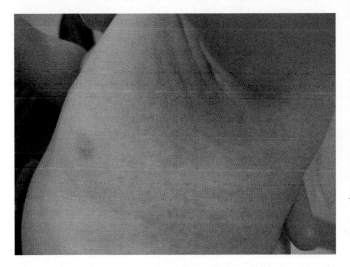

Unilateral laterothoracic exanthem (Fig. 6.19) is a papulosquamous disorder. Cases have been reported almost exclusively in Caucasian children, most children being 2–3 years in the largest series, with female to male ratios of 2:1. A case series of 48 children demonstrated 46 Caucasian children and only one Black and one Asian child. Lesions begin with small erythematous papules often with a pale halo, becoming eczematous plaques localized to the unilateral inner chest, arm, and axillae for 2 weeks, after which generalization occurs over the trunk and proximal extremities for 1–4 weeks. Resolution occurs rapidly thereafter. Given the rarity of such cases in individuals of color, and the relative paucity of papular pityriasis rosea in Caucasians, I have always

believed this may represent an atypical form of pityriasis rosea of Caucasian children. Association has been noted with a variety of viral infections including B-19 parvovirus and parainfluenza [19].

Lichen Planus (Figs. 6.20–6.23)

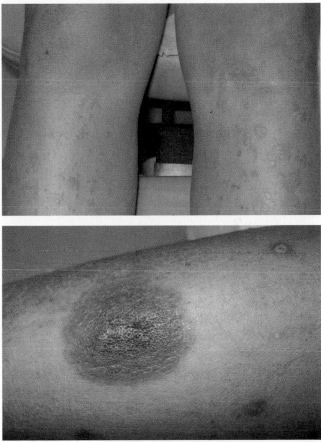

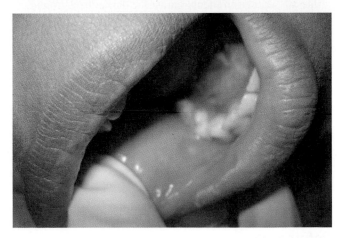

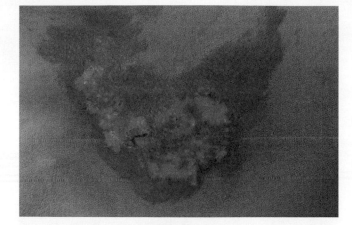

Lichen planus is an inflammatory disorder of unknown etiology that affects children, from school age through adolescence, with a mean age of 11.8 years and a 2:1 female to male ratio. In a recent analysis of pediatric cases at a single institution, 72% were African American as opposed to 21% of the background population. Twenty-two percent of children had oral lesions and 8% linear lesions. In the Caucasian child, purple pruritic plaques over the extremities are noted. Assorted infectious etiologies have been postulated and we have noted clustering of cases. Reports have shown that triggering of disease via HBV vaccination can occur in childhood [20]. In children of color, disease severity is often extensive and hypertrophic, necessitating oral corticosteroid therapy.

Lesions demonstrate purple, polygonal, planar papules. In Caucasian and Asian children, bright purple-red coloration is noted. Darker purple to violaceous lesions is noted in Hispanic children (Fig. 6.20). Anterior skin lesions are often hypertrophic in children of color. In the hypertrophic lesion pictured in Fig. 6.21, Wickham's striae, a network of light reticulate patterning is noted over the surface. Wickham's striae are more prominent against the darker background.

Oral lesions of lichen planus are less common in childhood than adulthood. Oral lesions are equally common in Caucasian and Black patients with lichen planus, but may be less common in Indian children [21]. In the Hispanic child shown, the oral mucosa has an erosive white plaque (Fig. 6.22).

Linear lichen planus (Fig. 6.23) is a disorder following the lines of Blaschko that has been reported primarily in Black, Hispanic/Latino, and Asian children. In my experience, lesions are often violaceous and hypertrophic in children of color. Response to high-potency topical corticosteroids is usually good [22].

References

 1. Silverberg NB (2009) Pediatric psoriasis: an update. Ther Clin Risk Manag 5:849–856

 2. Wu JJ, Black MH, Smith N, Porter AH, Jacobsen SJ, Koebnick C (2011) Low prevalence of psoriasis among children and adolescents in a large multiethnic cohort in southern California. J Am Acad Dermatol 65:957–964

 3. Chiam LY, de Jager ME, Giam YC, de Jong EM, van de Kerkhof PC, Seyger MM (2011) Juvenile psoriasis in European and Asian children: similarities and differences. Br J Dermatol 164:1101–1103

 4. Koebnick C, Black MH, Smith N, Der-Sarkissian JK, Porter AH, Jacobsen SJ, Wu JJ (2011) The association of psoriasis and elevated blood lipids in overweight and obese children. J Pediatr 159:577–583

 5. Abdel-Hamid IA, Agha SA, Moustafa YM, El-Labban AM (2003) Pityriasis amiantacea: a clinical and etiopathologic study of 85 patients. Int J Dermatol 42:260–264

 6. Hansted B, Lindskov R (1983) Pityriasis amiantacea and psoriasis. A follow-up study. Dermatologica 166:314–315

 7. Morris A, Rogers M, Fischer G, Williams K (2001) Childhood psoriasis: a clinical review of 1262 cases. Pediatr Dermatol 18:188–198

 8. Porto Ferreira C, Martins CJ, Issa PR, De Vasconcellos Carvalhaes de Oliveira R, Da-Cruz AM (2010) Psoriasis affects individuals of African descent and white Brazilians similarly. Actas Dermosifiliogr 101:230–234

 9. Gelfand JM, Stern RS, Nijsten T, Feldman SR, Thomas J, Kist J, Rolstad T, Margolis DJ (2005) The prevalence of psoriasis in African Americans: results from a population-based study. J Am Acad Dermatol 52:23–26

10. Shah SK, Arthur A, Yang YC, Stevens S, Alexis AF (2011) A retrospective study to investigate racial and ethnic variations in the treatment of psoriasis with etanercept. J Drugs Dermatol 10:866–872

11. Brazzelli V, Carugno A, Alborghetti A, Grasso V, Cananzi R, Fornara L, De Silvestri A, Borroni G (2011) Prevalence, severity and clinical features of psoriasis in fingernails and toenails in adult patients: Italian experience. J Eur Acad Dermatol Venereol. doi:10.1111/j.1468-3083.2011.04289.x

12. Wu Y, Lin Y, Liu HJ, Huang CZ, Feng AP, Li JW (2010) Childhood psoriasis: a study of 137 cases from central China. World J Pediatr 6:260–264

13. Al-Mutairi N, Manchanda Y, Nour-Eldin O (2007) Nail changes in childhood psoriasis: a study from Kuwait. Pediatr Dermatol 24:7–10

14. Tan E, Tay YK, Goh CL, Chin Giam Y (2002) The pattern and profile of alopecia areata in Singapore—a study of 219 Asians. Int J Dermatol 41:748–753

15. Sakata S, Howard A, Tosti A, Sinclair R (2006) Follow up of 12 patients with trachyonychia. Australas J Dermatol 47:166–168

16. Kalb RE, Bagel J, Korman NJ, Lebwohl MG, Young M, Horn EJ, Van Voorhees AS (2009) National Psoriasis Foundation. Treatment of intertriginous psoriasis: from the Medical Board of the National Psoriasis Foundation. J Am Acad Dermatol 60:120–124

17. Gündüz O, Ersoy-Evans S, Karaduman A (2009) Childhood pityriasis rosea. Pediatr Dermatol 26:750–751

18. Amer A, Fischer H, Li X (2007) The natural history of pityriasis rosea in black American children: how correct is the "classic" description? Arch Pediatr Adolesc Med 161:503–506

19. McCuaig CC, Russo P, Powell J, Pedneault L, Lebel P, Marcoux D (1996) Unilateral laterothoracic exanthem. A clinicopathologic study of forty-eight patients. J Am Acad Dermatol 34:979–984

20. Walton KE, Bowers EV, Drolet BA, Holland KE (2010) Childhood lichen planus: demographics of a U.S. population. Pediatr Dermatol 27:34–38

21. Handa S, Sahoo B (2002) Childhood lichen planus: a study of 87 cases. Int J Dermatol 41:423–427

22. Kabbash C, Laude TA, Weinberg JM, Silverberg NB (2002) Lichen planus in the lines of Blaschko. Pediatr Dermatol 19:541–545

Ichthyosis Vulgaris (Figs. 7.1–7.4)

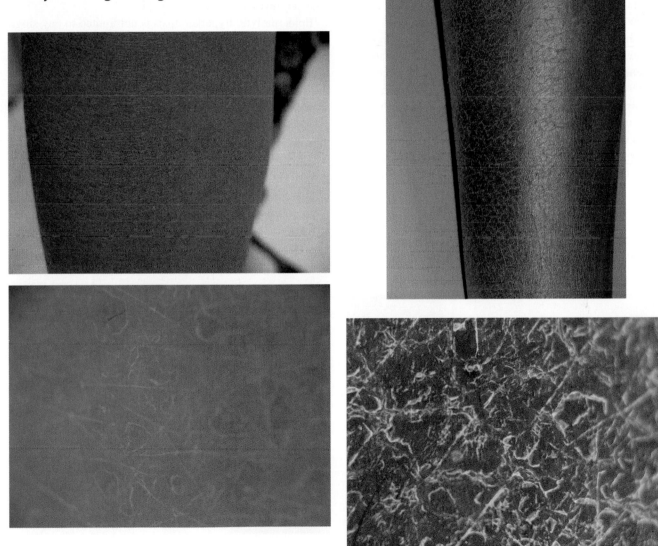

Ichthyosis vulgaris is the most common form of dry skin, inherited as an autosomal dominant trait due to mutations in filaggrin. Although estimates have suggested the prevalence at 1 in 250 individuals, the true incidence is likely far higher

N.B. Silverberg, *Atlas of Pediatric Cutaneous Biodiversity: Comparative Dermatologic Atlas of Pediatric Skin of All Colors*,
DOI 10.1007/978-1-4614-3564-8_7, © Springer Science+Business Media, LLC 2012

Table 7.1 Clinical features of ichthyosis vulgaris

Xerosis
Plate-like, irregular, fine scale over the extensor forearms and shins
More severe cases have scaling over the forehead (10.7% of Black atopics) and lower abdomen in infancy
Hyperlinear palms
Pruritus and/or atopic dermatitis can be features. Dermoscopy demonstrate prominent epidermal intercellular spaces and ragged cellular borders

since filaggrin polymorphisms are noted in upwards of 8% of the general population [1]. About 20% of atopic dermatitis patients have ichthyosis and the incidence of atopic dermatitis in the United States exceeds 10% [2], leaving at least 2% of children or 1 in 50 with ichthyosis vulgaris being a more likely disease estimate. Features of ichthyosis vulgaris are noted in Table 7.1.

The clinical appearance of ichthyosis vulgaris over the shins in a dark Asian child (Fig. 7.1) and the corresponding dermoscopy (Fig. 7.2) in this same child demonstrates the presence of retained keratinocytes with ragged borders.

Despite background pigmentation, the appearance of ichthyosis vulgaris in a Black child is easily noted as a dull, fine scale over the shins (Fig. 7.3). Dermoscopy demonstrates characteristic prominent intercellular spaces, with keratosis pilaris-like follicular changes (Fig. 7.4), demonstrating that these xerotic phenomena associated with atopic dermatitis can be concurrent. Dermoscopy may highlight the follicular features.

Epidermolytic hyperkeratosis (Fig. 7.5) (also called bullous congenital ichthyosiform erythroderma, bullous ichthyosiform erythroderma, or bullous congenital ichthyosiform erythroderma Brocq) is a rare autosomal dominant (rarely recessive) genodermatoses caused by mutations in keratins 1 or 10. There are reports of genetic transmission via gonadal mosaicism associated with solitary cutaneous epidermal nevi of epidermolytic hyperkeratosis histologic type [3]. In infancy lesions can be bullous in nature, gradually progressing to the adult phenotype of elephantine rugose thickening of the skin in the forehead and flexural extremities, as demonstrated in this teenage girl from the Dominican Republic. Therapies include topical keratolytics, therapy for bacterial overgrowth, and judicious usage of oral vitamin A derivates (higher dosages may aggravate the blistering tendency, even in older patients) [4].

Epidermolytic hyperkeratosis is not limited to any single race or ethnicity; however, this is one of the few conditions where the thickened skin can be at times darker in patients who are Caucasian than in children of color, where the color differences may not be as dramatic. Many children with this disorder appear dirty, and in fact bacteria and terra firma may complicate their skin appearance, irrespective of race and ethnicity.

Lamellar Ichthyosis (Figs. 7.6 and 7.7)

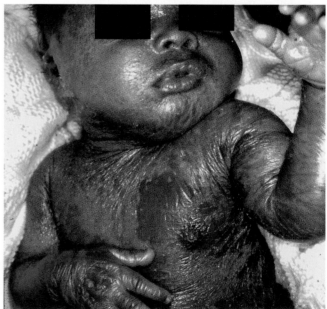

Epidermolytic Hyperkeratosis (Fig. 7.5)

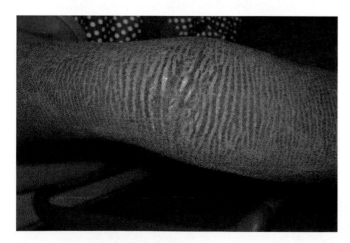

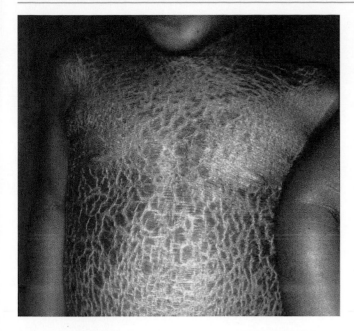

Lamellar Ichthyosis is an autosomal recessive genodermatosis caused by mutations primarily in transglutaminase 1 and less often in ALOXE3, ALOX12B, NIPAL4, and CYP4F22. Family history of consanguinity should be sought.

Children are often born with a collodion membrane (Fig. 7.6). Children will vary from self-healing in infancy to more-severe phenotypes including generalized plate-like scale or erythroderma with hyperkeratosis. It would appear that this ichthyosis affects individuals of all racial types similarly. Plate-like scales over the torso are particularly noticeable due to pigmentation in the Black patient pictured in Fig. 7.7. Table 7.2 demonstrates a diagnostic paradigm for diagnosing ichthyosis.

Congenital Ichthyosiform Erythroderma (Fig. 7.8)

Table 7.2 Diagnostic paradigm for ichthyoses [5]

Personal and family history
Onset of disease
Initial symptoms
Associated personal or family history of atopy (e.g., Netherton syndrome)
Consanguinity (recessive disorders)
History of hair growth
History of blistering (epidermolytic hyperkeratosis)
History of recurrent infections (e.g., *Staphylococcus aureus* in Netherton syndrome)
Neurological degeneration (e.g., Sjogren-Larsson)
Cryptorchidism (X-linked recessive ichthyosis) (mostly Caucasian patients, less so Hispanic and Asian; rare for African American) [6]
Hypohidrosis/heat intolerance
Developmental delays or mental retardation
Birth and in utero history: delayed rupture of membranes (X-linked recessive ichthyosis), shortened foot or debris in the amniotic fluid on 24 week ultrasound (Harlequin ichthyosis) [7]
Physical examination
Type and location of hyperkeratosis
Evaluations
Hair evaluation
In vivo hair dermoscopy or dermoscopy at 20× of cut hairs [8] (Can demonstrate trichothiodystrophy and Trichorrhexis invaginata of Netherton syndrome)
Biopsy for H and E, electron microscopy, immunoflourescence mapping
Blood cell counts, chemistries, complete metabolic panel
Steroid sulfatase levels, FISH for steroid sulfatase (X-linked recessive ichthyosis is primarily a disease of Caucasians, less so Asian and Hispanic; males only)
Genetic evaluation/genetic testing for specific suspected gene abnormalities (e.g., SPINK5 in Netherton syndrome)
Bacterial cultures of skin with odor or areas with rapid flairs or oozing

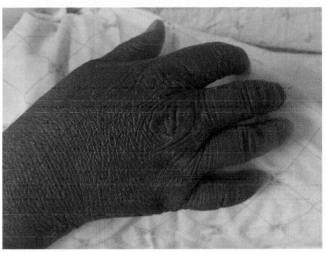

This 9-year-old Hispanic boy has congenital ichthyosiform erythroderma (Fig. 7.8) with notable generalized shiny brown scales, similar to lamellar ichthyosis over the distal extremities, as shown here, but fine erythema of the face. The scales are especially dark in children of color. Like many children of his age, he is heat-intolerant and prone to dehydration due to abnormal skin barrier; however such an issue will also be seen in some ectodermal dysplasia syndromes. Emollients and keratolytic agents topically may be helpful. Oral retinoids will correct the skin defect; however, usage in girls of child bearing age should be used cautiously due to risk of pregnancy.

Harlequin Ichthyosis (Fig. 7.9)

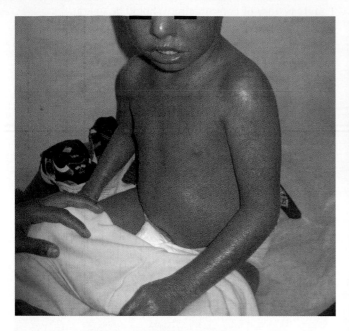

Harlequin ichthyosis is an autosomal recessive ichthyosis caused by severe gene mutations of the ABCA12 gene, in which children are born with thick shiny encasements over the entire body causing restrictive skin disorders, including ectropion, eclabium and shortened feet, visible on prenatal ultrasound. Although death was nearly universal 100 years ago, early introduction of acitretin and good neonatal intensive care has resulted in children surviving infancy.

These children go on to have a severe congenital ichthyosiform erythroderma phenotype as they age, as noted in Fig. 7.9. Consanguinity is often noted in parents, and many cases reported come from areas of the world where consanguinity is not uncommon, e.g., Middle East. The shiny membranes and the underlying erythema differ little by skin tone, race, and ethnicity.

Porokeratosis (Figs. 7.10–7.14)

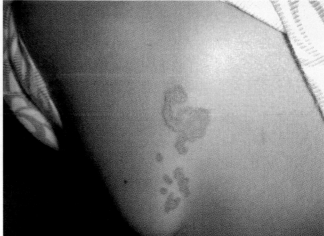

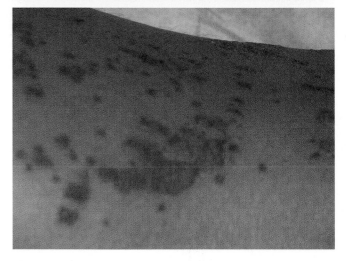

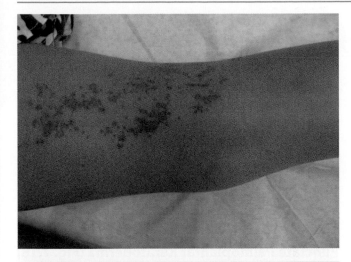

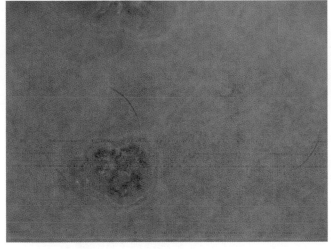

demonstrates dilated pores on dermoscopy with keratinous plugs as noted in this Hispanic girl. Furrow ink test will confirm blockage of ductal structures [10].

Linear porokeratosis (Figs. 7.12 and 7.13), which may represent a loss of heterozygosity may be either linear lesions with raised borders or linear hyperkeratotic lesions, following the lines of Blascko. Dermoscopy demonstrates a cornoid lamella around the lesion which is a raised tract around the lesion and in this case central follicular plugging which is cribriform (Fig. 7.14). Similar to lichen planus, linear porokeratosis in Black children (Fig. 7.13) is often hypertrophic in nature. Application of topical trichloracetic acid 50–75% resulted in 50% reduction in lesion thickness.

Palmoplantar Keratoderma (Figs. 7.15–7.17)

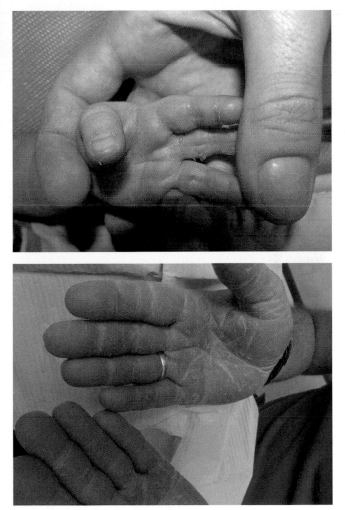

Porokeratosis is an uncommon disorder of keratinization. Lesions appear as sharply demarcates, annular plaques, often with hyperkeratosis. The raised border has a cornoid lamella histologically. Five types have been described, classic porokeratosis of Mibelli, disseminates superficial porokeratosis (the actinic type is not seen in childhood), porokeratosis Palmaris et plantaris disseminate, linear porokeratosis, and punctate porokeratosis. Disseminated superficial actinic porokeratosis, because lesions are sun-induced, is rare in Black patients [9].

In the 8-year-old Asian girl shown in Fig. 7.10, porokeratosis of Mibelli was diagnosed by biopsy, despite the lack of family history. Good response was noted to mid-potency topical corticosteroids and topical calcipotriene 0.005%. Lesions are notably darker in the punctuate porokeratosis shown in a Hispanic child in Fig. 7.11. Porokeratosis

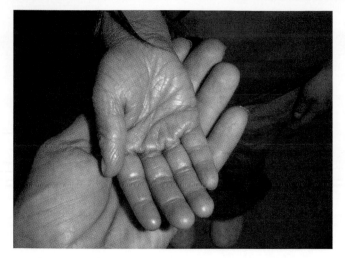

Table 7.3 Diagnosing palmoplantar keratodermas [15]

Personal and family history
Onset of disease
Initial symptoms
Presence or absence of associated personal or family history of heart disease, esophageal tumors (e.g., Howel-Evans), oral plaques (e.g., Olmsted syndrome), gingivitis (e.g., Papillon-Lefevre), keratitis (e.g., Tyrosinemia type II)
Consanguinity (recessive disorders)
Country of origin (e.g., Greece for Naxos disease) or state of origin (Virginia for Richner Hanhart disease)
History of hair growth (e.g., PPK with atrichia, wooly hair in Naxos disease)
History of blistering (Dowling Meara epidermolysis bullosa simplex)
History of odor (e.g., Mal de Meleda)
History of deafness (e.g., Vohlwinkel)
History of digital amputation (e.g., Sybert) or limb deformity (e.g., Huriez)
Presence of nail abnormalities (e.g., hyperkeratosis in pachyonychia congenital)
Hyperhidrosis
Developmental delays or mental retardation (e.g., Richner Hanhart)
Physical examination
Type and location of keratoderma
Associated features
Extension of keratoderma
Evaluations
Hair evaluation
Biopsy for H and E (e.g., epidermolytic hyperkeratosis in Vorner type), electron microscopy, immunoflourescence mapping
Blood cell counts, chemistries, complete metabolic panel
Genetic evaluation/genetic testing for specific suspected gene abnormalities
Bacterial cultures of skin with odor or areas with rapid flairs or oozing

Palmoplantar keratodermas are a group of disorders in which the skin of the palms and soles are thickened. This can result in a hyperkeratotic plaque or shiny thickened skin. This infant with Unna-Thost variety (Fig. 7.15) has a father (Fig. 7.16) and a grandmother with palmoplantar hyperkeratosis

and no medical problems other than some hyperhidrosis. Histologically, these cases do not demonstrate epidermolytic hyperkeratosis.

Palmoplantar keratodermas (Fig. 7.17) with epidermolytic hyperkeratosis histology, i.e., epidermolytic palmoplantar keratoderma, which is caused by a mutation in keratin 9, has been described to have some different genetic mutations as the cause in Italian (Caucasian) [11], Chinese [12], and Japanese [13] patients, with some overlap due to a genetic "hot spot" in position 162 (R162W) of the gene (Terrinoni).

A basic schema of how to classify palmoplantar keratodermas is listed in Table 7.3.

Punctate Palmoplantar Keratoderma (Fig. 7.18)

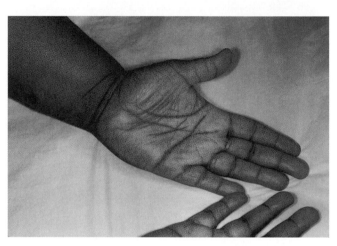

As the palms and soles are relatively lighter than other portions of the body, keratodermas of Black patients often demonstrate a yellow thickened skin. When hyperpigmented areas are noted on the palms and soles lesions may be warts, lichen planus, or punctuate keratodermas, either porokeratotic type typified by small papules with underlying hyperpigmented pits or dells in Black patients or Buschke-Fischer-Brauer disease, typified by circumscribed thickened areas. Keratosis punctata of the palmar creases is a variant noted in Fig. 7.18, which is common in Black/African patients, but exceedingly rare in Caucasians [14].

References

1. Chen H, Common JE, Haines RL, Balakrishnan A, Brown SJ, Goh CS, Cordell HJ, Sandilands A, Campbell LE, Kroboth K, Irvine AD, Goh DL, Tang MB, van Bever HP, Giam YC, McLean WH, Lane EB (2011) Wide spectrum of filaggrin-null mutations in atopic dermatitis highlights differences between Singaporean Chinese and European populations. Br J Dermatol 165:106–114
2. Shaw TE, Currie GP, Koudelka CW, Simpson EL (2011) Eczema prevalence in the United States: data from the 2003 National Survey of Children's Health. J Invest Dermatol 131:67–73

3. Paller AS, Syder AJ, Chan YM, Yu QC, Hutton E, Tadini G, Fuchs E (1994) Genetic and clinical mosaicism in a type of epidermal nevus. N Engl J Med 331:1408–1415

4. Morais P, Mota A, Baudrier T, Lopes JM, Cerqueira R, Tavares P, Azevedo F (2009) Epidermolytic hyperkeratosis with palmoplantar keratoderma in a patient with KRT10 mutation. Eur J Dermatol 19:333–336

5. Oji V, Traupe H (2009) Ichthyosis: clinical manifestations and practical treatment options. Am J Clin Dermatol 10:351–364

6. Craig WY, Roberson M, Palomaki GE, Shackleton CH, Marcos J, Haddow JE (2010) Prevalence of steroid sulfatase deficiency in California according to race and ethnicity. Prenat Diagn 30(9): 893–898

7. Suresh S, Vijayalakshmi R, Indrani S, Lata M (2004) Short foot length: a diagnostic pointer for harlequin ichthyosis. J Ultrasound Med 23:1653–1657

8. Silverberg NB, Silverberg JI, Wong ML (2009) Trichoscopy using a handheld dermoscope: an in-office technique to diagnose genetic disease of the hair. Arch Dermatol 145:600

9. Doherty CB, Krathen RA, Smith-Zagone MJ, Hsu S (2009) Disseminated superficial actinic porokeratosis in black skin. Int J Dermatol 48:160–161

10. Uhara H, Kamijo F, Okuyama R, Saida T (2011) Open pores with plugs in porokeratosis clearly visualized with the dermoscopic furrow ink test: report of 3 cases. Arch Dermatol 147: 866–868

11. Terrinoni A, Cocuroccia B, Gubinelli E, Zambruno G, Candi E, Melino G, Girolomoni G (2004) Identification of the keratin K9 R162W mutation in patients of Italian origin with epidermolytic palmoplantar keratoderma. Eur J Dermatol 14:375–378

12. Chen XL, Xu CM, Cai SR, Chen CY, Zhang XN (2009) Prenatal diagnosis of epidermolytic palmoplantar keratoderma caused by c. T470C (p.M157T) of the keratin 9 gene in a Chinese kindred. Prenat Diagn 29:911–913

13. Kon A, Itagaki K, Yoneda K, Takagaki K (2005) A novel mutation of keratin 9 gene (R162P) in a Japanese family with epidermolytic palmoplantar keratoderma. Arch Dermatol Res 296: 375–378

14. Peñas PF, Rios-Buceta L, Sánchez-Pérez J, Dorado-Bris JM, Aragüés M (1994) Keratosis punctata of the palmar creases: case report and prevalence study in Caucasians. Dermatology 188:200–202

15. Lucker GP, Van de Kerkhof PC, Steijlen PM (1994) The hereditary palmoplantar keratoses: an updated review and classification. Br J Dermatol 131:1–14

Eczematous Diseases

Atopic Dermatitis ("Eczema")

Atopic dermatitis is the most common skin condition seen in a pediatric dermatology clinic in developed nations, with symptomatology especially common in the 2–5 year age range. Atopic dermatitis is defined as a relapsing or chronic pruritic skin disorders, primarily of early onset, with typical distribution in infancy on the face and extensors, in childhood on the flexural areas and over the hands and feet in adults. Seventy percent of children will have a family history of atopy and many of the children themselves will have comorbid atopy (e.g., asthma, allergic rhinitis and/or conjunctivitis, atopic dermatitis), especially when a parent has asthma. Food allergies should be suspected in children with history of food-induced flares, extensive disease with poor response to therapy, and in children with family history of food allergy.

Allergen patterns should be kept in mind based on the child's ethnicity. While milk, egg, and soy are the leading allergens in most studies worldwide; Middle Eastern children have early sesame exposures and are more at risk for such allergies [1]. Asian children are exposed to shellfish and peanuts early on (6–12 months) and rates of allergy are 39% and 27%, respectively, in children tested [2]. When suspected, avoidance of oral and topical food allergens is essential.

Atopic dermatitis affects children of all races and ethnicities; however, differences exist in the incidence of atopic dermatitis by race and ethnicity, in the clinical features, in the response to therapies (both prescription and over-the-counter) and in the associated stigmata and general health problems that arise in association with atopic dermatitis.

Children who are Black are 1.7 times more likely to have atopic dermatitis than Caucasian children in the United States. Asian and Black children are more likely to have medical visits for atopic dermatitis than Caucasian children [3]. Almost 75% of atopic dermatitis cases seen in a pediatric dermatology clinic in Miami were Black children [4]. The east coast of the United States has the highest prevalence of cases, exceeding 11.5% in most states of the region [5]. The prevalence of atopic dermatitis in the Hispanic population of South America appears to be 11.3%; however, data on the incidence of minor criteria in Hispanic children is lacking and is therefore not included in Table 8.1 [23]. Filaggrin mutations are highly associated with atopic dermatitis in all ethnicities and races, with palmar hyperlinearity and keratosis pilaris being noted espccially in Asian children with filaggrin mutations [11].

Clinical features notably variable by race or ethnicity include the increased presence of Dennie-Morgan folds, lichenoid changes and perifollicular accentuation in Asian and Black children, higher incidence of associated keratosis pilaris and pityriasis alba in Indian children with atopic dermatitis (Nagaraja), high incidence of comorbid ichthyosis vulgaris in Asian children (Chen), and greater food and environmental intolerance amongst Caucasian children (Bohme). Differences exist between ethnic and racial groups in the specific mutations in the filaggrin gene [24]. Minor criteria may be quite uncommon in children under the age of 2 years, especially Scandinavian children (Bohme). Finally, Caucasian children have greater transepidermal water loss, but African American children demonstrated reductions in ceramide, resulting in abnormal skin barriers in both cases, but by different mechanisms [25].

N.B. Silverberg, *Atlas of Pediatric Cutaneous Biodiversity: Comparative Dermatologic Atlas of Pediatric Skin of All Colors*, DOI 10.1007/978-1-4614-3564-8_8, © Springer Science+Business Media, LLC 2012

Table 8.1 Atopic dermatitis diagnostic criteria and presence of the criteria by race or ethnicity[a]

Diagnostic criteria [6, 7]	White/Caucasian [8–10]	Asian [11–14]	Indian/South Asians [8, 11, 15–18]	Black [11, 19]
Dermatitis affecting the flexural surfaces in adults and the face or extensors in infants	8.7–13.7% (by visualization/by report)	1.8–5.3% point prevalence	0.83% (point prevalence)–6.64% incidence	38.5% extensor elbows ages 0–3 years 56.8% flexural elbows ages 4–18 years 14.2–24.8% (by visualization/by report)
Personal or family history of atopy	Personal: respiratory allergies (46%); asthma (9.87%) Family: mothers 72.4%; fathers (65.5%)	Personal: 39.8–69.3% with other forms of atopy Allergic rhinitis 59.8%; asthma 28.2% Family history: 56–66.7% (Wisuthsarewong)	Personal: 18.5% other forms of atopy Family history: 40%	Personal: 52.3% with other forms of atopy Family history: 41.7%
Incidence	8.7% AD (16.5% at 2 years; 4.7% adults) 22.5% Atopy	13.3–21% AD	7.4–16% AD	4.7–16.3%
Minor criteria				
Early age of onset	15.8% by 3.5 years	49% by 10 years 65.7% by 2 years	31–53.12%	40.6–51.3% (42 weeks/10 years)
Keratosis pilaris	4–5% at 2 years	7.1–29.2%	14.8–33%	16.7%
Ichthyosis	9% of Europeans carry filaggrin mutations [20]	8,19.2, 24.1, 51.3%	4, 34.3%	21.4%
Hyperlinear palms	No data	31.5–49.1%	23–24.8%	51.8%
Hand and foot dermatitis	Hand (28%)	25.4–36.1%	Hand (9%) Foot (7.6%)	20.1%
Perifollicular accentuation (syn. papular lichenoid changes)	1% at 2 years	47.2–64.6%	39%	Papular lichenoid 54.1%
Circumoral pallor	No data	40.8%	26%	No data
Pityriasis alba (%)	6	25, 28.7, 53.1	14.3–34	13.1
Cheilitis (%)	1	8.3–63.1	3–10.5	4
Infraorbital darkening	0% at 2 years (Swedish)	39.2–50%	12%	54.3%
Infraorbital folds [21] (Dennie-Morgan lines)	2–3% (2 years); 25% in mixed age populus	21.3–52.3%	39.5–63%	49.2%
Recurrent conjunctivitis	No data	12%	14%	1.3%
Anterior neck folds	1% at 2 years	46.9–72.2%	6%	No data
Nipple eczema	No data	4.6–13.8%	No data	7.5%

Feature				
Triggers including: foods (F), emotional factors (Em). environmental factors (En) and irritants (IR e.g., wool (W), solvents (So), sweat (Sw), humidity (H))	87% (En) 39% (F) 34% (Sw)	36.1% (F) 24.1 % (W) 13.9% (So) 77.8% (Sw)	41% (W,So) 50–66.7% (W) 26.7% (Sw) 19.0% (F) 6.7% (So)	3.5% (F) 1.3% (Em/stress) 5.5% (En/grass) 30.8% (En/dry season) 39.3% (Sw) 38.3% (H) 3.9% (drug)
Susceptibility to cutaneous viral (V), fungal (F), and bacterial (B) infections	1–2% at 2 years	19.4%	36–80%	2.9% (V) 37% (F) 41.7% (B) Scabies (9.9%)
Immediate skin-test reactivity	29–72%	23.9–41.2%	No data	No data
White dermographism (%)	3	18.5–37.7	40	7.4
Raised serum IgE	41%	60%		Raised peripheral blood eosinophils 51% [22]

aPruritus and relapsing dermatitis are required for diagnosis and should be universal; therefore, they are not included in this chart; dry skin, keratoconus. Impaired cell-mediated immunity and anterior subcapsular cataracts have been removed from minor criteria due to lack of reported data

Atopic Dermatitis—Infantile (Fig. 8.1)

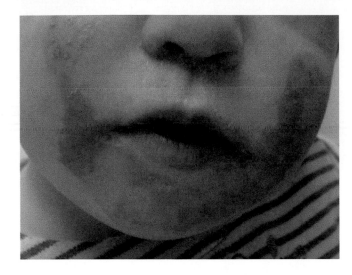

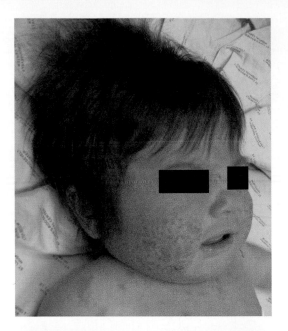

Infantile atopic dermatitis is the typical variant with facial (Fig. 8.1) and flexural distribution. The disease is marked in infancy by extreme erythema, serosanguineous discharge, and comorbid seborrheic dermatitis. Initiation of what I term the HAE skin care regimen using bath-hydration followed by agent application (where needed) and emolliation (HAE) are essential to care and maintenance of the skin in atopic dermatitis [26] (Table 8.2).

Facial Atopic Dermatitis (Figs. 8.2– 8.4)

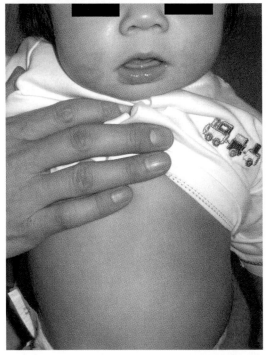

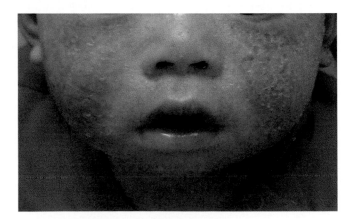

Individuals of Asian descent generally have greater facial sensitivity (Fig. 8.2). A recent study demonstrated low barrier maturation and weak skin barrier in East Asians and to some extent Caucasians with atopic dermatitis [28]. Facial sensitivity starts with infantile irritant contact dermatitis and in genetically predisposed individuals, atopic dermatitis and turns into facial redness in response to cosmetics and emollients in adulthood. In my experience, usage of gentle skin care products such as low pH, fragrance-free agents are essential in this community. In the child pictured in Figs. 8.3 and 8.4, institution of oral cephalexin and topical hydrocortisone 2.5% ointment with good skin care result in lesion resolution over a 2-week time period.

Table 8.2 Skin care of children with atopic dermatitis

Intervention	Intermittent or continuous	Specific instructions
Gentle skin care: fragrance-free soaps or syndets	Continuous	Cleanse skin using fragrance-free, gentle cleansers; Syndets and fragrance-free soaps (mixed with emollients)
Gentle skin care: bathe daily (hydrate)	Intermittent	Soak in bathtub when skin disease is active
		Limit bathing to 15 min or less
		Avoid very hot bathwater
Gentle skin care: emolliate	Continuous	Lotions for summer
		Creams, oils, petrolatum, and glycerin products for winter (patients from the Near East and Middle East may have preference for oil-based emollients)
		Discourage purchase of cocoa butter or other agents from outdoor flea market vendors (sterility of product cannot be ascertained)
		Discourage usage of raw botanicals. Usage of raw botanical agents may unwittingly expose children to fragrance or allergens such as pollen
Gentle skin care: enhanced emollients	Intermittent	Enhanced moisturizers with ceramides, colloidal oatmeal, and filaggrin by-products may improve moisturization (in children of darker skin tones (IV–VI) with concurrent ichthyosis vulgaris, petrolatum overlying ceramide-enhanced moisturizers may be required due to a combination of lower ceramide content than other races and thicker stratum corneum)
Gentle skin care: sift fabrics	Continuous	Cotton clothing is ideal for children with skin problems
Gentle skin care: fragrance-free, dye-free detergents	Continuous	Detergents without added fragrance or dyes
Gentle skin care: bath additives	Intermittent	Addition of oils or colloidal oatmeal to the bath for rapid relief of pruritus
		Addition of bleach (see header on "Special Situations: Recurrent Bacterial Superinfection")
Topical medicaments: "Devices"	Intermittent to continuous	Topical "Devices," i.e., emollients with anti-inflammatory additives (e.g., glycerrhetinic acid, ceramide, PEA)
		To be used adjunctively to other topical agents to reduce the need for topical corticosteroids
Topical medicaments: topical corticosteroids	Intermittent	Low potency (class 5–7) for facial and intertriginous lesion, for infants and for large surface area
		Mid-potency products applied after bath to affected lesions for moderate to severe disease
		Soak and slather techniques-generalized application after bath for extensive body surface areas
Topical medicaments: topical calcineurin inhibitors[a]	Intermittent	Topical calcineurin inhibitors[a] for topical corticosteroid failures, intertriginous, genital or facial disease and/or pityriasis alba
		Pimecrolimus 1% cream for mild to moderate atopic dermatitis, ages 2 years and over
		Tacrolimus 0.03% ointment for moderate to severe atopic dermatitis ages 2–15 years
		Tacrolimus 0.1% ointment for moderate to severe atopic dermatitis ages 16 and older or for children of color who have fair but incomplete response to 0.03% ointment (consider tacrolimus 0.1% in children of color skin types IV–VI, who have been shown to have greater resistance to tacrolimus 0.03%)
Pruritus care/relief of sleep disturbance	Intermittent	Oral antihistamines at bedtime
		Wet pajamas covered by dry pajamas
		Silver-impregnated silk pajamas
Therapy of severe atopic dermatitis: oral immunosuppressants	Intermittent	Oral immunosuppressants (All require screening blood counts, chemistries, and liver function testing)
For large body surface area, erythroderma and/or intractable symptomatology		Cyclosporine A (not for patients with renal disease)
		Requires additional monitoring of blood pressure and renal function
		Mycofenelate mofitil
		Methotrexate (not for patients with liver disease)

(continued)

Table 8.2 (continued)

Intervention	Intermittent or continuous	Specific instructions
Therapy of severe atopic dermatitis: ultraviolet light therapy	Intermittent	Ultraviolet light therapy (not for patients with lupus or other forms of photosensitivity; Initiate soak and slather of medications prior to avoid heat- or sweat-based flares with UV therapy)
		Narrowband UVB (Best for ages 7 and over) [27]
For large body surface area, erythroderma and/or intractable symptomatology		Generalized (for extensive disease)
		Hand-foot unit (for palmoplantar disease)
Special situation: recurrent bacterial superinfection of atopic dermatitis	Intermittent	Bacterial culture of nares and affected area
		Oral antibiotics 1–2 weeks
		Mupirocin for the 3N's: Nares, Navel, Nails (optional: anus)
		Bleach Bathes (1/4 cup bleach in half full tub; soak 15–20 min twice-weekly)
		Household usage of ethyl alcohol handrubs
		Culture and treat household Staph carriers
Special situation: food allergies	Continuous and intermittent care	Avoidance of the allergen both as an ingested food and in topical preparations
		When suspected in early infancy, empiric shifting of formula from milk or soy-based to alimental formulations may be needed
		Prescribe epinephrine auto-injector for anaphylactic reactions (age-appropriate dosage)
		Refer for allergy testing for high body surface areas, intractable disease, history of allergic-type symptoms with food ingestion and strong family history of food allergy (especially anaphylaxis)
Seasonal care: winter	Intermittent	Vitamin D supplementation, 400 IU all skin tones
		Cool-mist humidifier
Seasonal care: summer	Intermittent	Fans and air conditioning
		Misting fans to cool child down
		Usage of insect repellants to avoid mosquito allergy-induced flares (DEET 3–5%, picardin)
		Fragrance-free sunscreens

Modified from Silverberg NB (2010) Pediatric dermatology in children of color. Access Dermatol

[a]Topical calcineurin inhibitors have a black-box warning on their label that states they are no for children under the age of 2 years, and they may be linked to lymphomas or skin cancers. While these linkages have not been proven, patients have to be informed of possible risk when usage is intended long-term

Infantile Atopic Dermatitis and Hypopigmentation (Fig. 8.5)

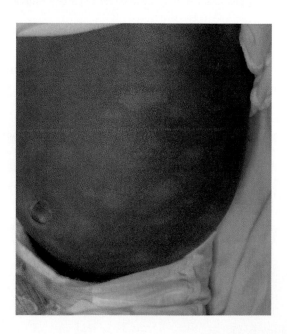

Infantile atopic dermatitis is bright red in the Caucasian and Asian infant, while being complicated by extensive hypopigmentation in Black children in infancy (Fig. 8.5), especially when complicated by comorbid seborrheic dermatitis. Black children with atopic dermatitis have a greater reduction as a racial or ethnic group in skin ceramide content [29]. In my experience, a two-step emolliation process using a ceramide-based product followed by petrolatum may be needed to correct severe xerosis in this grouping [28].

Follicular Atopic Dermatitis (Figs. 8.6–8.8)

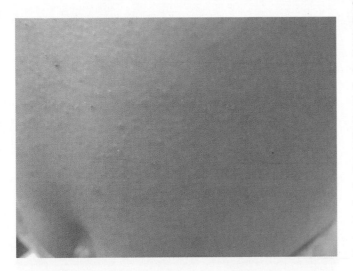

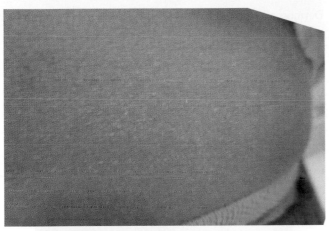

Follicular eczema is more common in children of color. Despite the lack of erythema in follicular eczema in children of color, this variant is extremely pruritic. Hence erythema scores alone may not be reflective of severity of atopic dermatitis in children of color [30]. Flares may be proceeded by mild follicular prominence, followed by extreme pruritus and associated eczematous alterations such as excoriations, erythema, and lichenification. Follicular eczema is rarer in Indian children, but when it occurs, perifollicular erythema and or pallor can be noted, the latter being a feature not usually noted in most ethnic groupings (Fig. 8.7).

Follicular eczema is exceedingly common in Black children, as shown in Fig. 8.8. Although atopic dermatitis is less commonly follicular by nature in Caucasians, this variant can be noted in Caucasians (Fig. 8.6). Particularly when the follicular prominence is noted over the abdomen, consideration of possible comorbid contact allergy (most commonly nickel) is of concern.

The management is similar in all ethnicities and races, except that thicker emollients are needed for darker children. Although literature is lacking on the subject, in my experience, follicular eczema in Black children is often resistant to low-potency corticosteroids and age-appropriate calcineurin inhibitors (0.03%) and at time requires prescription of Class 2 or 3 corticosteroid agents or tacrolimus 0.1% ointment in some children to address the follicular component [29]. There is a need for short-term usage of higher potency products and careful monitoring of lesions to avoid atrophy, given the lack of lichenification of the skin in this group of children.

Flexural Atopic Dermatitis (Figs. 8.9 and 8.10)

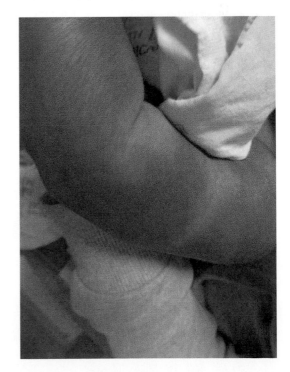

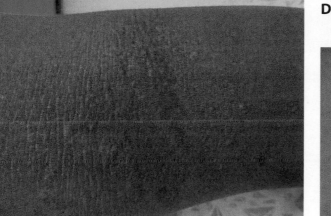

Dermoscopy of Atopic Dermatitis (Fig. 8.11)

Hispanic and African American children often experience significant pigmentary alterations due to atopic and seborrheic dermatitis. In infancy and early childhood, hypopigmentation prevails (Fig. 8.9). However, with maturation of the pigmentary system of the skin, hyperpigmentation will become more common. When hypopigmentation is noted in a child of type I–III skin, it is often due to the lack of tanning noted in atopic lesions, creating a relative hypopigmentation as the lesion fades.

Flexural atopic dermatitis is the most common site of mid-childhood; however, lesion type varies by race and ethnicity. Caucasian children have erythema and excoriations prevailing. Older children, especially Black children, experience hyperpigmentation associated with lichenification of the flexural areas from chronic rubbing and scratching (Fig. 8.10). In this African American boy with flexural atopic dermatitis, hyperpigmentation and extensive lichenification are noted, with minimal excoriations, despite months of active scratching. It is important when counseling parents to recommend limitation of therapy to a few weeks at a time and only for active lesions, or what I term the 4 Rs—redness, raised lesions, roughness, or rasca (Spanish for scratching). Specifically, in children of color it is advisable to caution parents to avoid therapy of smooth, asymptomatic skin that has pigmentary alterations.

Dermoscopy of atopic dermatitis (Fig. 8.11) demonstrates dilated vasculature and xerotic changes of the epidermis (prominent intercellular spaces). When associated ichthyosis vulgaris is noted, ragged keratinocyte edges are noted as well on dermoscopy. Improvements in skin are noted after emolliation.

Lichen Simplex Chronicus—Extensor Surfaces African American (Figs. 8.12 and 8.13)

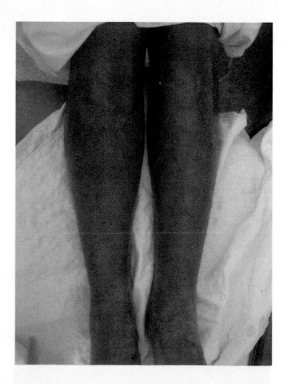

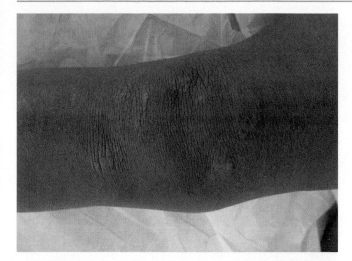

Lichenification over the shins is not uncommon in African American teenagers (Fig. 8.13) who wear high-top sneakers. The friction seems to exacerbate the disease locally. Other causes of shin lichenification in older children and adolescents are sweat-induced flares under shin guards for soccer and contact allergies (irritant or allergic) secondary to agents ranging from nylons to shaver strips.

Juvenile Plantar Dermatosis (Fig. 8.14)

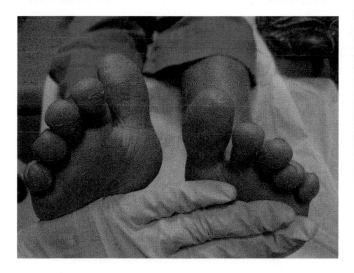

Hyperhidrosis of the feet is more common in Caucasian children (personal observation). When a child with atopic dermatitis (especially boys aged 3–14 years) and hyperhidrosis wears occlusive footwear (e.g., plastic shoes) in summer, the sweat trapping can initiate a shiny dermatitis on the underside of the toes and balls of the feet, sparing the interdigital webs, and termed juvenile plantar dermatosis. Half of all the children with this illness will have atopic dermatitis and some children will have concurrent staphylococcal or micrococcal overgrowth [31].

In these children, cutaneous hydration with thick emollients and dimethicone creams is needed and natural socks and shoes (cotton, canvas, and leather) in order to absorb excess sweat, the disease trigger. Cycling shoes every 48 h to allow for complete dryness of footwear may be beneficial in both this condition and in cases of recurrent tinea pedis, a dermatophyte infection of the plantar foot. Forty-one percent of cases will have an associated contact allergen including rubber adhesives and potassium dichromate [32].

Superinfected Atopic Dermatitis (Fig. 8.15)

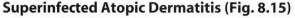

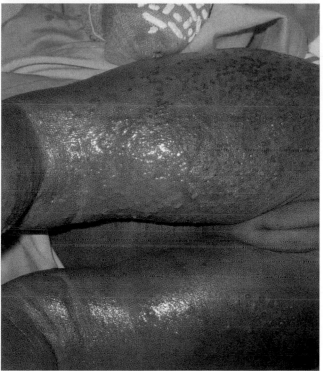

Atopic dermatitis patients are more prone to colonization, overgrowth, and infection with *Staphylococcus aureus* [33]. Although resistant species may be less common culture isolates in children with atopic dermatitis [34], nevertheless, *S. aureus* can make atopic dermatitis flare spread and can result in abscess formation or deep tissue infection if left untreated. This child with atopic dermatitis is grossly infected with *S. aureus* (Fig. 8.15). Recurrent infections were noted due to colonization of the nares. Oral cephalexin was beneficial in clearing crusts, some pruritis and open sores, but concurrent topical corticosteroids were needed to clear underlying inflamed lesions of atopic dermatitis. Usage of clindamycin or trimethoprim sulfamethoxazole (required in *methicillin-resistant S. aureus*-endemic areas) would be an alternative therapeutic option.

Erythroderma and Generalized Lichenification African American (Figs. 8.16 and 8.17)

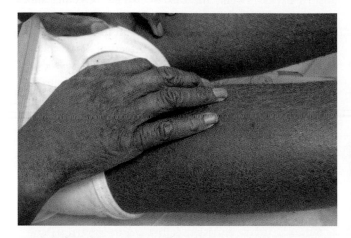

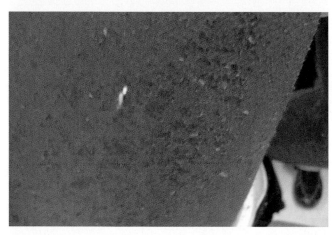

When atopic dermatitis is chronic and severe, generalization of disease develops, which is termed erythroderma (Fig. 8.16). In a Caucasian individual bright red erythema can be noted. In Black children a generalized hyperpigmented thickening and fine erythema (Fig. 8.17) head to toe may be noted to be superimposed.

Branny Scale in a Black Infant with Atopic Dermatitis (Fig. 8.18)

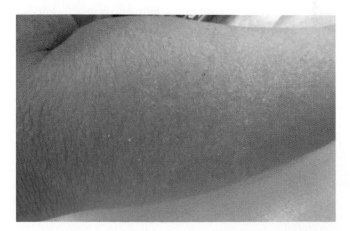

When children are infected with *S. aureus* on their atopic dermatitis, I often note a generalized fine branny scale with peeling. The scales may be pigmented in a child of color, as noted here. Oral antibiotics are required, in addition to atopic dermatitis care. If fever or malaise is noted, intravenous therapy may be required to treat the infection.

Lichen Planus-Like Atopic Dermatitis/Lichenoid Atopic Dermatitis (Figs. 8.19 and 8.20)

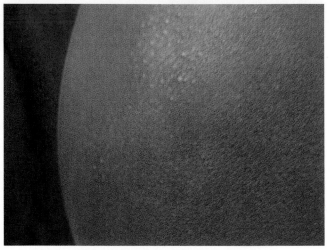

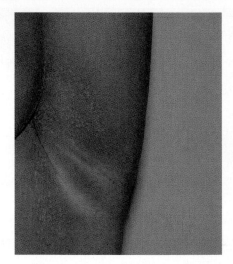

This variant of atopic dermatitis presents in Black children with lichenoid papules on the extensor surfaces. Biopsy demonstrates the typical spongiotic dermatitis of atopic dermatitis. Children respond to topical agents similarly to atopic dermatitis. In this 15-year-old African American boy (Fig. 8.19) who has had lesions since the age of 7 years (Fig. 8.20), pruritic papules occur in the axillae forearms, wrists, and over the ankles. Oral erosive lesions occur in response to trauma in this boy, but biopsy demonstrates spongiotic dermatosis [35]. Lichenoid lesions have been described in 54.1% of African Blacks with atopic dermatitis [19].

Dermatitis Erythema Nuchae (Fig. 8.21)

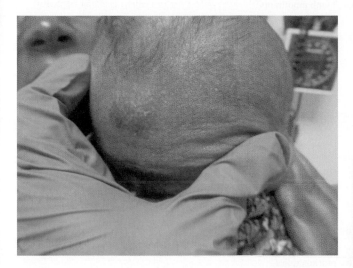

For children with nevus simplex over the nuchal region, atopic dermatitis can localize overlying this area or accentuate there, resulting in a very violaceous plaque (Fig. 8.21). Parents have to be warned that the violaceous hue will persist even when the eczematous changes resolve. This reaction is more commonly noted in Caucasian than African American infants, due to the greater incidence of nevus simplex in Caucasians.

Eczema Herpeticum (Fig. 8.22)

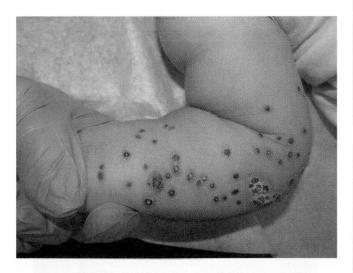

In children with atopic dermatitis, risk of infection is greater due to reduced amount and lack of ability to induce production of cathelicidins [36] and beta defensins [37]. Herpes simplex virus (Fig. 8.22) can spread rapidly, as noted in this child with eczema herpeticum. Note the vesicles are red to purple. Lesions are often less discrete in individuals of color, presenting with greater erosive lesions with scalloped borders as is noted in the child in Fig. 8.16. Pain and rapid onset

are clues to the diagnosis. One clinical issue that obscures diagnosis of eczema herpeticum is comorbid impetigo, which is common in children with eczema herpeticum. Concurrent antibiotic therapy can aid in clearance and lesional resolution. When extensive erosions are present in an atopic child, especially when discomfort is present, bacterial and viral cultures are required.

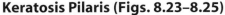

Keratosis Pilaris (Figs. 8.23–8.25)

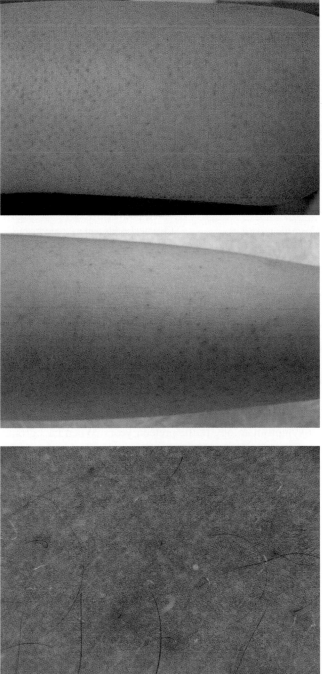

Table 8.3 Instructions for patients with keratosis pilaris

Gentle skin care	Fragrance-free, gentle cleansers
	Syndets and fragrance-free soaps (mixed with emollients)
	Gentle bathing (hydrate)
	Bathtub soaks when skin disease is active
	Limit bathing to 15 min or less
	Avoid very hot bathwater
	Moisturizers (Emolliate)
	Lotions for summer
	Creams, oils, petrolatum and glycerin products for winter (patients from the Near East and Middle East may have preference for oil-based emollients)
	Enhanced moisturizers with ceramides, colloidal oatmeal, and filaggrin by-products may improve moisturization (in children of darker skin tones (IV–VI) with concurrent ichthyosis vulgaris, petrolatum overlying enhanced moisturizers may be required)
	Discourage purchase of cocoa butter or other agents from outdoor flea market vendors (sterility of product cannot be ascertained)
	Soft fabrics, esp. cotton
	Detergents without added fragrance or dyes
	Bath additives
	Addition of oils or oatmeal to the bath for pruritus relief
	Addition of bleach (see header on recurrent infections)
	Usage of raw botanical agents may unwittingly expose children to fragrance or allergens such as pollen
Loufa sponge	Gently exfoliate reachable skin (2–3 gentle passes)
Enhanced emollients	Keratolytic emollients (e.g., Urea 20% or less, lactic acid 5–12%)
	Emollients with hydrating additives (e.g., sunflower oils)
Prescription exfoliants	Prescription of higher strength exfoliants including retinoids (e.g., tretinoin, adapalene, tazarotene) can improve skin appearance
Cosmetic procedures	Chemical peels and microdermabrasion can be used for rapid improvements of appearance

Keratosis pilaris is a cutaneous form of xerosis where lack of exfoliation at the hair follicle is noted over the cheeks, upper arms, upper thighs, and/or buttocks. While occasionally associated with cardiofaciocutaneous syndrome in its severe scarring form (ulerythema oophyrogenes) [38], keratosis pilaris is usually genetic, being inherited in an autosomal dominant fashion (Table 8.3).

Onset in the toddler years is common, with a second peak of symptomatology in the preteen years. When background erythema is noted, it is termed Keratosis pilaris rubra faciei. Mean age of onset of the latter is 5 years of age. While many children outgrow facial lesions in puberty, disease persists over the upper arm and upper thigh into adulthood. Obesity will exacerbate disease at any age.

Keratosis pilaris in Caucasian and Hispanic children manifests with erythema of the follicular orifice as noted in Fig. 8.24. In Black children, hyperpigmentation of the follicular orifice is noted as seen in Fig. 8.25. Dermoscopy of the patient in Fig. 8.25 demonstrates fine erythema/dilated vasculature and retention hyperkeratosis around the hair follicles (Fig. 8.26). The dermoscopic picture shows both keratosis pilaris and ichthyosis vulgaris on the legs. A resultant pattern

of pigmented inter-keratinocyte spaces and follicular hyperkeratosis and pigmentation is noted.

Keratosis Pilaris Rubra Faciei (Figs. 8.26–8.28)

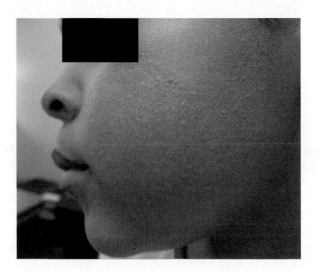

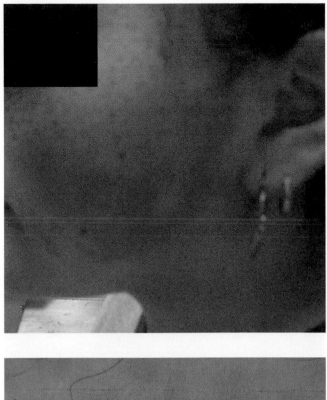

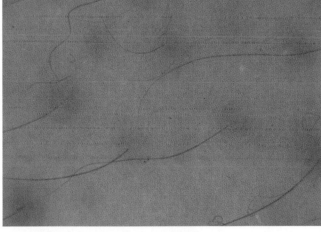

Like the usage of pulsed dye laser for port wine stains, postinflammatory hyperpigmentation can occur.

Dennie Morgan Caucasian (Fig. 8.29)

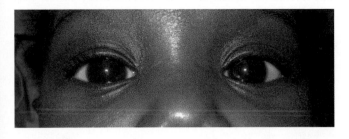

The Dennie Morgan fold (Fig. 8.29) is a benign infraorbital fold under the eye that begins lateral to the medial canthus. Dennie Morgan folds are common in individuals with atopic dermatitis; however, they are common in all patients of color, especially Black children, even in the absence of a history of atopy. Twenty-five to twenty-seven percent of children with atopic dermatitis manifest a Dennie Morgan fold. Forty-nine percent of Indian and Black children and 25% of Caucasian children will have an infraorbital crease [21]. Infraorbital darkening is also common in Caucasian children with atopic dermatitis, sometimes termed allergic shiners.

Nipple Eczema (Fig. 8.30)

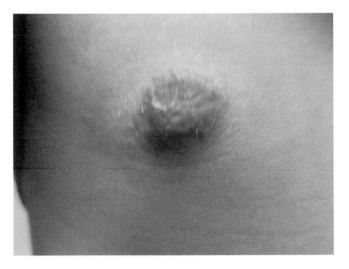

Keratosis pilaris rubra faciei is typified by erythema ranging from mild (Fig. 8.26) to severe (Fig. 8.27). This form is not generally seen in African American children. Facial keratosis pilaris is common in Caucasian and Hispanic children, but uncommon for Asian and African American children. In children of color, pigmentation of the follicle can accompany disease. On dermoscopy (Fig. 8.28) of the patient from Fig. 8.27 perifollicular erythema and edema of the follicular orifice are noted.

When erythema is severe, judicious usage of pulsed dye laser can reduce facial erythema in these individuals.

Nipple eczema is a minor criterion of atopic dermatitis which is more prevalent in Asian and Indian children. This photo (Fig. 8.30) depicts a male Asian baby with nipple dermatitis in association. Though under-reported, atopic dermatitis of the nipples and genitalia are common, the latter having onset after potty training. These types of eczema can persist into adulthood. Consequently cotton undershirts or bras may always be required.

Hand Eczema (Fig. 8.31)

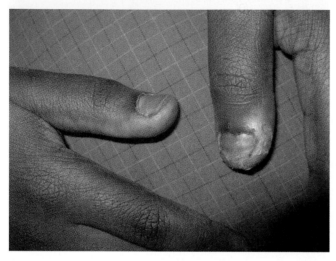

One of the minor features of atopic dermatitis is hand eczema (Fig. 8.31). Hand eczema may be the adult form of atopic dermatitis precipitated by wetwork, allergens and irritants, but is by no means limited to adults and may occur in nonatopics. A clinical mimic is acrodermatitis of Hallopeau, a form of psoriasis of the distal digits.

In a recent Spanish cohort, about 50% of children with hand eczema had allergic contact dermatitis to preservatives (e.g., Kathon CG) and fragrance, with 76.2% being relevant allergies. This results in a third of all pediatric hand eczemas being caused or exacerbated by allergic contact dermatitis. As a result, gentle skin care using fragrance-free agents and reduced-preservative formulations may aid in clearance of active disease in childhood [39]. Usage of cotton gloves under vinyl gloves for wetwork can further protect the skin.

In my experience, Black children experience more eczema in the periungual space and this area needs to be emolliated liberally.

Infantile Seborrheic Dermatitis (Figs. 8.32–8.34)

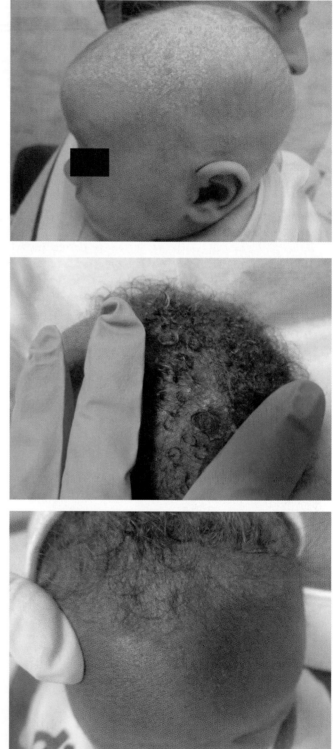

Seborrheic dermatitis, known in the vernacular as cradle cap, is an inflammatory dermatosis caused by early sebaceous gland activity and reaction to colonization with *Malasssezia* species. In Caucasian children (Fig. 8.32), seborrheic dermatitis is a yellow-pink greasy scale over the crown, accompanied by intertriginous plaques with maceration. Caucasian scale can get so severe as to form a crusted helmet of hyperkeratosis. In children of color, hyperkeratosis can range from flesh-colored scales to a helmet of slightly lighter, macerated skin encrusted over the crown.

Black and Hispanic children with seborrheic dermatitis will experience extensive pigmentary alterations, usually hypopigmentation, accompanying their seborrheic dermatitis (Figs. 8.33 and 8.34).

Gentle skin care, hydration, and mild corticosteroids often clear this condition without sequelae. When hypopigmentation occurs, it is not caused by topical corticosteroids; however, usage of milder topical agents is best to avoid exacerbation of the pigmentary disturbance. Dandruff shampoos can aid in clearance. Sterile oil (medical grade, not food grade oils) can be used to soften the hyperkeratosis to aid in removal. Borage oil and ceramide-based emollients may be helpful to aid in clearance of symptoms as well.

Many children with extensive seborrheic dermatitis will go on to have atopic dermatitis. It is unclear whether the *Malassezia* species is the triggering event for atopic dermatitis or whether these children have intrinsic barrier defects predisposing to both conditions.

Allergic Contact Dermatitis (Figs. 8.35–8.40)

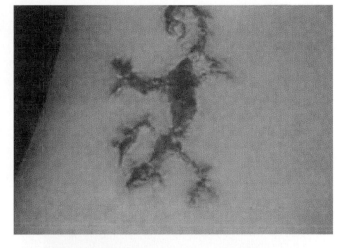

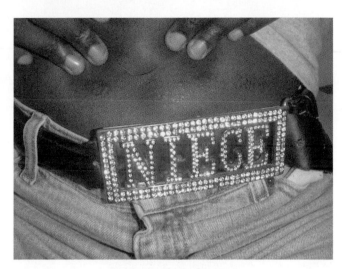

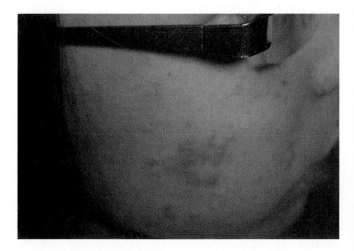

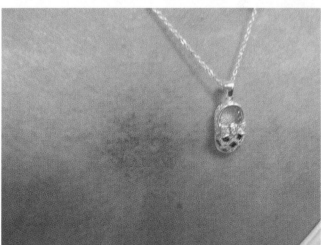

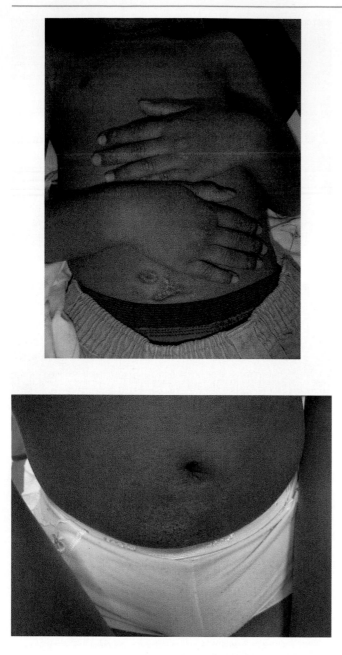

Allergic contact dermatitis is a universal pattern of cutaneous type IV, cell-mediated immunity. Universal contact allergens are allergens to which all individuals can react if contact is achieved. These include poison ivy (uruchiol) (Fig. 8.35) and the medically used agents dinitrochlorobenzene (which is mutagenic on the Ames test) and squaric acid (nonmutagenic on the Ames test). Rarely are cutaneous allergens reported to be more common by race; however trends toward greater cobalt allergy in individuals of color have been reported [40].

Contact dermatitis can be caused by casual exposures to allergens or by introduction through a wound. The patient shown in Fig. 8.36 developed an allergic contact reaction to his henna tattoo of a gecko, gotten on vacation. The allergenic culprit in this case is paraphenylenediamine. As henna tattoos are most commonly used by individuals from India and the Middle East, consideration of this allergy in individuals of these backgrounds is important when looking at scalp dermatoses in individuals who color their hair.

Comparative data on the incidence of allergic contact dermatitis by race and ethnicity has not been published for children, leaving this as a large gap in knowledge; however, no differences exist in small-scale studies [41].

Nickel allergy (Figs. 8.37–8.39) is universally the most common allergen along with fragrance in any and all racial and ethnic groupings. Early and aggressive exposures seem to initiate sensitization. For this reason the European Union has recently created legislation limiting production of metal clothing with extensive nickel content. In the United States, many children's clothing stores have initiated reductions in nickel content, which has begun to limit the buttonfly reaction. However, belt buckles, especially the large white metal type often worn by African American and Hispanic children have created a style-induced surge of infraumbilical disease in this grouping [42]. Early sensitization to nickel can occur through early piercing or via exposures such as snaps and belt buckles.

Caucasian children experience more eczematous changes with allergic contact dermatitis reactions Fig. 8.36, resulting in thick erythematous plaques, often abrupt or recurrent in onset. Lesions are often angulated based on exposure sites. However, with nickel allergy, the movement of nickel through clothing and against the dynamic skin results in blurred edges (Figs. 8.37 and 8.38).

Hispanic children with allergic contact dermatitis often have extensive hyperpigmentation in the region and notable follicular-based lesions (Fig. 8.40), which are common to children of color. Nickel allergies run a spectrum of severity from mild erythema to chronic lichenification to generalized hypersensitivity (ID reaction) with widespread pruritus and lichenoid eczematous plaques of the extensor surfaces. The id reaction is often misdiagnosed because it does not occur in the areas of contact with nickel, but rather at distant sites. When extensor extremity dermatitis is noted, examination of the abdomen for a primary site of contact dermatitis to nickel may aid in diagnosis.

Black and African American children may demonstrate mottled hyperpigmentation and lichenification in the infraumbilical region and extensor extremities (Figs. 8.39 and 8.40). Testing jewelry for nickel using the Dimethylglyoxime test allows patients to purchase clothing without nickel (Table 8.4).

Table 8.4 Nickel avoidance techniques

Avoid all nonessential metal purchases
Stainless steel, sterling silver (92.5%+), high-content yellow gold (18K+/75%+)
For metal belts, belt buckles and costume jewelry including ball and chain necklaces and watch backs, test with dimethylglyoxime test prior to purchase
Do not hold cell phone against face
For owned items with nickel, apply two coats of clear nail polish liberally twice-weekly or after each wash
Reduce oral nickel ingestion by avoiding canned goods, chocolate, nuts, soy, kippered herring, oats, peas, rye, red kidney beans. Legumes, tea, and whole wheat [43]

Table 8.5 Top allergens in childhood [44] and where they are found

Nickel (belts, buttonflies, cell phones, jewelry, canned foods)
Cobalt chloride (jewelry, belts)
Neomycin sulfate (antibacterial preparations)
Potassium dichromate (shoes, cement-noted in juvenile plantar dermatosis) [45]
Fragrance (personal care products)
Cocapropamidyl betaine (shampoos)
p-tert-butylphenol formaldehyde resin (personal care products, makeup, ready to wear clothing)
Thimerosal[a] (vaccines, antibacterial agents)
Wool alcohols (emollients)
Rubber additives (shoes, as noted in juvenile plantar dermatosis) [2]
Methylchloroisothiazolinone/methylisothiazolinone

[a]Vaccine-related sensitization will be reduced due to withdrawal of this agent from many vaccines

Cell Phone Allergy (Fig. 8.41)

Lichen Striatus (Figs. 8.42–8.44)

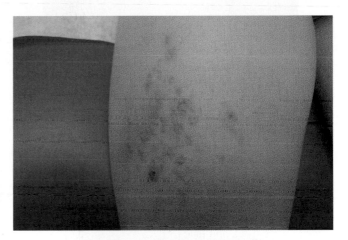

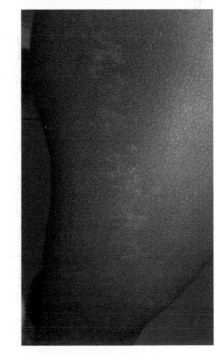

Nickel allergic contact dermatitis can be caused by extensive jewelry exposure, however, the most common accessory on the arm of teenagers, irrespective of race or ethnicity, is a cell phone (Fig. 8.41). Metallic covers can contain nickel, resulting in contact dermatitis along the jawline. The lesions will often be circular based upon the contact surface exposure when the phone is held between the jaw and the shoulder (Table 8.5).

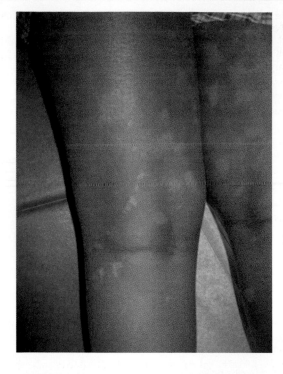

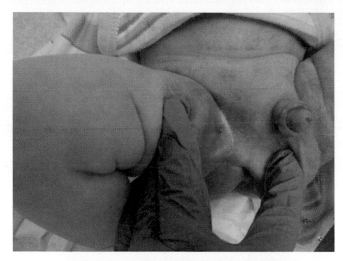

Lichen striatus is an asymptomatic linear dermatitis occurring along the lines of Blaschko. Lichen striatus occurs in two phases. The first 6–24 months is phase 1, typified by dermatitis with small papules extending from distal to proximal, usually along the limbs. Resolution (Phase 2) is marked by hypopigmentation which is most obvious in Caucasian children when tanned. A recent review of 24 episodes in children from Spain showed that most children have solitary lesions with 2/3 of cases occurring on the extremities, followed by the trunk and face [39].

In a Caucasian child, lesions are erythematous papules with dermoscopic features of dilated vasculature (similar to atopic dermatitis). In the Asian child in Fig. 8.42, the inflammatory phase of lichen striatus can be seen. Prolonged postinflammatory hyperpigmentation is noted after flattening. Papules may be lightly pigmented in Asian and Hispanic children with lichen striatus, but in general, hypopigmentation (Fig. 8.43) prevails in children of skin types IV and over. Surrounding hypopigmentation is notable in the patient in Fig. 8.43, despite lack of therapy. It is unclear whether prompt initiation of topical corticosteroids can prevent hypopigmentation in these individuals.

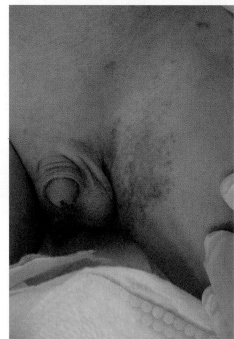

Lichen striatus in Black children often presents with linear grouped hypopigmented pinpoint papules along the lines of Blaschko. Postinflammatory hypopigmentation that is cosmetically significant is often seen in Phase 2 in darker children (Fig. 8.44). Resolution of this hypopigmentation is enhanced with excimer or narrowband UVB treatments, but spontaneous resolution is expected in a few years with or without therapy.

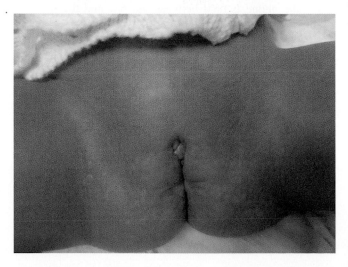

Candidal diaper dermatitis is universal to children in diapers. However Caucasian children, manifest bright red erythema and satellite pustules (Fig. 8.45), while children of color may have more violaceous erythema and pigmentary incontinence with hypopigmentation as a sequela of resolution (Figs. 8.45 and 8.46).

Diaper dermatitis of the irritant form is most common and is usually caused by altered pH in the diaper area; these areas may develop secondary infection with *Candida* species. In these cases, mild, broad erythema of the groin and intertriginous folds is complicated by shiny maceration. In Caucasian children, salmon pink plaques may be noted, while Hispanic and Black children will manifest more violaceous erythema (Fig. 8.47) and postinflammatory hypopigmentation.

Irritant Contact Dermatitis—Facial (Fig. 8.48)

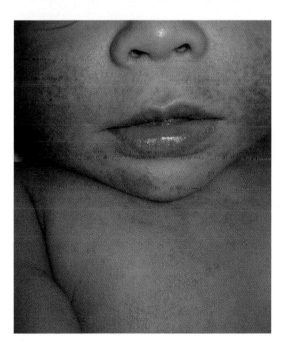

Excess salivary secretion (drool) due to teething, messy eating, and mouth breathing are some of the reasons that infants develop irritant contact dermatitis of the face (Fig. 8.48). Disease occurs in all races and ethnicities, but Asian and Caucasian children appear to have the most sensitive facial skin. Usage of syndets to clean the face and frequent emollient application to the face as a skin protectant can aid in retention of healthy facial skin until exacerbants like drooling fade with age. A brief recurrence can be noted at age 2 years with the eruption of the second year molars.

References

1. Aaronov D, Tasher D, Levine A, Somekh E, Serour F, Dalal I (2008) Natural history of food allergy in infants and children in Israel. Ann Allergy Asthma Immunol 101:637–640
2. Chiang WC, Kidon MI, Liew WK, Goh A, Tang JP, Chay OM (2007) The changing face of food hypersensitivity in an Asian community. Clin Exp Allergy 37:1055–1061
3. Horii KA, Simon SD, Liu DY, Sharma V (2007) Atopic dermatitis in children in the United States, 1997-2004: visit trends, patient and provider characteristics, and prescribing patterns. Pediatrics 120:e527–e534
4. Schachner L, Ling NS, Press S (1983) A statistical analysis of a pediatric dermatology clinic. Pediatr Dermatol 1:157–164
5. Shaw TE, Currie GP, Koudelka CW, Simpson EL (2011) Eczema prevalence in the United States: data from the 2003 National Survey of Children's Health. J Invest Dermatol 131:67–73
6. Hanifin JM, Rajka G (1980) Diagnostic features of atopic dermatitis. Acta Derm Venereol (Stockh) 92:44–47
7. Rothe MJ, Grant-Kels JM (1996) Diagnostic criteria for atopic dermatitis. Lancet 348:769–770
8. Williams HC, Pembroke AC, Forsdyke H, Boodoo G, Hay RJ, Burney PG (1995) London-born black Caribbean children are at increased risk of atopic dermatitis. J Am Acad Dermatol 32:212–217
9. Purvis DJ, Thompson JM, Clark PM, Robinson E, Black PN, Wild CJ, Mitchell EA (2005) Risk factors for atopic dermatitis in New Zealand children at 3.5 years of age. Br J Dermatol 152:742–749
10. Böhme M, Svensson A, Kull I, Nordvall SL, Wahlgren CF (2001) Clinical features of atopic dermatitis at two years of age: a prospective, population-based case-control study. Acta Derm Venereol 81:193–197
11. Chen H, Common JE, Haines RL, Balakrishnan A, Brown SJ, Goh CS, Cordell HJ, Sandilands A, Campbell LE, Kroboth K, Irvine AD, Goh DL, Tang MB, van Bever HP, Giam YC, McLean WH, Lane EB (2011) Wide spectrum of filaggrin-null mutations in atopic dermatitis highlights differences between Singaporean Chinese and European populations. Br J Dermatol 165:106–114
12. Wisuthsarewong W, Viravan S (2004) Diagnostic criteria for atopic dermatitis in Thai children. J Med Assoc Thai 87:1496–1500
13. Lee HJ, Cho SH, Ha SJ, Ahn WK, Park YM, Byun DG, Kim JW (2000) Minor cutaneous features of atopic dermatitis in South Korea. Int J Dermatol 39:337–342
14. Tay YK, Khoo BP, Goh CL (1999) The epidemiology of atopic dermatitis at a tertiary referral skin center in Singapore. Asian Pac J Allergy Immunol 17:137–141
15. Nagaraja KAJ, Dhar S, Singh S (1996) Frequency and significance of minor clinical features in various age-related subgroups of atopic dermatitis in children. Pediatr Dermatol 13:10–13
16. Dhar S, Banerjee R (2010) Atopic dermatitis in infants and children in India. Indian J Dermatol Venereol Leprol 76:504–513
17. Patel JK, Vyas AP, Berman B, Vierra M (2010) Incidence of childhood dermatosis in India. Skinmed 8:136–142
18. Wahab MA, Rahman MH, Khondker L, Hawlader AR, Ali A, Hafiz MA, Ansari NP (2011) Minor criteria for atopic dermatitis in children. Mymensingh Med J 20:419–424
19. Nnoruka EN (2004) Current epidemiology of atopic dermatitis in south-eastern Nigeria. Int J Dermatol 43:739–744
20. Smith FJ, Irvine AD, Terron-Kwiatkowski A, Sandilands A, Campbell LE, Zhao Y, Liao H, Evans AT, Goudie DR, Lewis-Jones S, Arseculeratne G, Munro CS, Sergeant A, O'Regan G, Bale SJ, Compton JG, DiGiovanna JJ, Presland RB, Fleckman P, McLean WH (2006) Loss-of-function mutations in the gene encoding filaggrin cause ichthyosis vulgaris. Nat Genet 38(3):337–342

21. Williams HC, Pembroke AC (1996) Infraorbital crease, ethnic group, and atopic dermatitis. Arch Dermatol 132:51–54
22. Levin ME, Le Souëf PN, Motala C (2008) Total IgE in urban Black South African teenagers: the influence of atopy and helminth infection. Pediatr Allergy Immunol 19:449–454
23. Solé D, Mallol J, Wandalsen GF, Aguirre V, Latin American ISAAC Phase 3 Study Group (2010) Prevalence of symptoms of eczema in Latin America: results of the International Study of Asthma and Allergies in Childhood (ISAAC) Phase 3. J Investig Allergol Clin Immunol 20:311–323
24. Hsu CK, Akiyama M, Nemoto-Hasebe I, Nomura T, Sandilands A, Chao SC, Lee JY, Sheu HM, McLean WH, Shimizu H (2009) Analysis of Taiwanese ichthyosis vulgaris families further demonstrates differences in FLG mutations between European and Asian populations. Br J Dermatol 161:448–451
25. Gupta J, Grube E, Ericksen MB, Stevenson MD, Lucky AW, Sheth AP, Assa'ad AH, Khurana Hershey GK (2008) Intrinsically defective skin barrier function in children with atopic dermatitis correlates with disease severity. J Allergy Clin Immunol 121:725–730.e2
26. Kiken DA, Silverberg NB (2006) Atopic dermatitis in children, part 1: epidemiology, clinical features, and complications. Cutis 78:241–247
27. Veith W, Deleo V, Silverberg N (2011) (2011) Medical phototherapy in childhood skin diseases. Minerva Pediatr 63:327–333
28. Muizzuddin N, Hellemans L, Van Overloop L, Corstjens H, Declercq L, Maes D (2010) Structural and functional differences in barrier properties of African American, Caucasian and East Asian skin. J Dermatol Sci 59:123–128
29. Hanifin JM, Ling MR, Langley R, Breneman D, Rafal E (2001) Tacrolimus ointment for the treatment of atopic dermatitis in adult patients: part I, efficacy. J Am Acad Dermatol 44:S28–S38
30. Ben-Gashir MA, Hay RJ (2002) Reliance on erythema scores may mask severe atopic dermatitis in black children compared with their white counterparts. Br J Dermatol 147:920–925
31. Gibbs NF (2004) Juvenile plantar dermatosis. Can sweat cause foot rash and peeling? Postgrad Med 115(6):73–75
32. Darling MI, Horn HM, McCormack SK, Schofield OM (2011) Sole dermatitis in children: patch testing revisited. Pediatr Dermatol. doi:10.1111/j.1525-1470.2011.01550.x
33. Nada HA, Gomaa NI, Elakhras A, Wasfy R, Baker RA (2012) Skin colonization by superantigen-producing Staphylococcus aureus in Egyptian patients with atopic dermatitis and its relation to disease severity and serum interleukin-4 level. Int J Infect Dis 16:e29–e33
34. Matiz C, Tom WL, Eichenfield LF, Pong A, Friedlander SF (2011) Children with atopic dermatitis appear less likely to be infected with community acquired methicillin-resistant Staphylococcus aureus: the San Diego experience. Pediatr Dermatol 28:6–11
35. Allen HB, Jones NP, Bowen SE (2008) Lichenoid and other clinical presentations of atopic dermatitis in an inner city practice. J Am Acad Dermatol 58:503–504
36. Wollenberg A, Räwer HC, Schauber J (2011) Innate immunity in atopic dermatitis. Clin Rev Allergy Immunol 41:272–281
37. Hata TR, Kotol P, Boguniewicz M, Taylor P, Paik A, Jackson M, Nguyen M, Kabigting F, Miller J, Gerber M, Zaccaro D, Armstrong B, Dorschner R, Leung DY, Gallo RL (2010) History of eczema herpeticum is associated with the inability to induce human β-defensin (HBD)-2, HBD-3 and cathelicidin in the skin of patients with atopic dermatitis. Br J Dermatol 163:659–661
38. Marqueling AL, Gilliam AE, Prendiville J, Zvulunov A, Antaya RJ, Sugarman J, Pang ML, Lee P, Eichenfield L, Metz B, Goldberg GN, Phillips RJ, Frieden IJ (2006) Keratosis pilaris rubra: a common but underrecognized condition. Arch Dermatol 142:1611–1616
39. Toledo F, Silvestre JF, Cuesta L, Latorre N, Monteagudo A (2011) Usefulness of skin-prick tests in children with hand eczema: comparison with their use in childhood and adult eczema. Actas Dermosifiliogr 102:429–438
40. Ruff CA, Belsito DV (2006) The impact of various patient factors on contact allergy to nickel, cobalt, and chromate. J Am Acad Dermatol 55:32–39
41. Jacob SE, Herro EM, Sullivan K, Matiz C, Eichenfield L, Hamann C (2011) Safety and efficacy evaluation of TRUE TEST panels 1.1, 2.1, and 3.1 in children and adolescents. Dermatitis 22:204–210
42. Silverberg NB, Licht J, Friedler S, Sethi S, Laude TA (2002) Nickel contact hypersensitivity in children. Pediatr Dermatol 19:110–113
43. http://www.dormer.com/physicians/html/nickel_allergies.htm
44. Simonsen AB, Deleuran M, Johansen JD, Sommerlund M (2011) Contact allergy and allergic contact dermatitis in children—a review of current data. Contact Dermatitis 65:254–265
45. Darling MI, Horn HM, McCormack SK, Schofield OM (2011) Sole dermatitis in children: patch testing revisited. Pediatr Dermatol. 2011 Aug 19. doi:10.1111/j.1525-1470.2011.01550.x. [Epub ahead of print] PubMed PMID: 21854421

Photosensitivity

Photosensitivity is a spectrum of medical conditions that cause increased response to light sources ranging from the visible spectrum to ultraviolet light. Photosensitivity in early childhood can be a result of normally thin, underpigmented infantile skin, circulating antibodies (e.g., neonatal lupus erythematosus), medication ingestion (e.g., anticonvulsants), and poor ability to repair one's skin after ultraviolet damage occurs.

Photosensitivity can be associated with a variety of medications used in childhood. Topical medicaments associated with photosensitivity include all the topical retinoid agents (adapalene, tazarotene, and tretinoin) in all concentrations, as well as alpha and beta hydroxy acids. While photosensitivity is more notable in lighter children, no race or ethnicity is spared. Phototoxic erythema is more likely with Caucasians and Hispanics in my practice; however, Black children who take these medications can certainly experience phototoxic erythema and tanning with prolonged sun exposure. As a result, usage of sunprotection on a daily basis is essential for all retinoid-users.

Photosensitivity of the skin (as opposed to photosensitive seizure activity) is common with childhood anticonvulsants including carbamazepine, oxcarbazene, phenytoin, and valproic acid; however, the clinician has to be careful to consider the possibility of a hypersensitivity reaction which can be more prominent in a photodistribution [1]. Another class of oral medications that are associated with childhood photosensitization is the oral antibiotics including demeclocylcine, doxycycline, minocycline, and trimethoprim-sulfamethoxazole, commonly used in acne sufferers.

A rare photosensitivity that is drug induced in children is naproxen-induced pseudoporphyria, a reaction reported primarily in Caucasian children of Fitzpatrick phototypes I and II who are treated with naproxen for juvenile rheumatoid arthritis. Blistering and fragility can persist for 4–6 months after drug discontinuation. Facial blistering in this condition can cause scarring, which persists for 5 or more years. Ibuprofen may also cause pseudoporphyria [2].

Neonatal Lupus (Figs. 9.1–9.3)

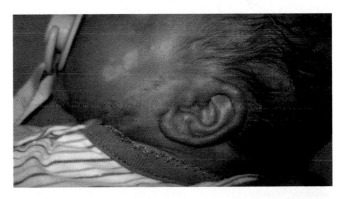

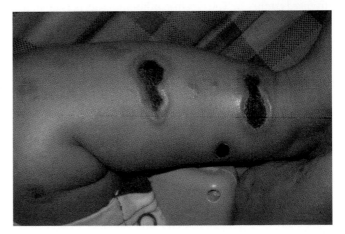

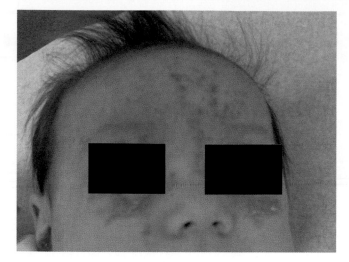

Table 9.1 Work-up of suspected neonatal lupus [4]

Cardiac: echocardiogram, EKG (64.7% with cardiac changes)
For mother and child: ANA, anti-Ro (SS-A), anti-La (SS-B), and U1 RNP antibodies (N.B. It is my experience that mothers may have anti-La antibodies with negative ANA, therefore, the full panel is needed when suspicion is high)
Complete blood count with differential (35.3% of infants with hematological changes)
Complete metabolic profile (esp. liver function tests) (52.9% with hepatobiliary changes)
Full skin examination and mucous membrane examination (70.6% with cutaneous changes)
Biopsies of suspicious lesions: for histopathology and/or immunofluorescence

Neonatal lupus is a form of lupus in which the autoimmune antibodies are transplacentally transferred from mother to child. Causative antibodies include anti-Ro (SS-A), anti-La (SS-B), and anti-U1RNP antibodies. Although the antibodies are transferred prenatally, lesions can be present at birth or begin months later, after sun exposure. Lesions are annular erythematous plaques, similar to that seen in subacute cutaneous lupus, and usually over the head and neck (Fig. 9.1) but erosions and scarring can be seen that behave and heal more like discoid lesions. Raccoon eyes due to atrophic periocular lesions and facial telangiectasias can be noted as well (Fig. 9.2).

In the Asian infant in Fig. 9.3, lesions were noted on the calves after the child went outside in shorts at 3 months of age. As is common, this mother was unaware that she had Sjogren's syndrome with positive SS-B antibodies. Cardiac evaluation is needed, as anti-La antibodies affect the cardiac conduction system development and pacemakers may be needed. When U1RNP antibodies are the only type, cardiac disease is unlikely. The electrocardiogram was normal in this patient and blood counts as well as liver function tests were normal as well. Careful sun protection and topical corticosteroids aided in lesion clearance, but discoloration and atrophic scarring were noted in areas of prior erosions.

Women of color are at greater risk of systemic lupus erythematosus. Black, Hispanic, and Asian women are far more likely than Caucasian women to develop lupus [3]. Consequently, neonatal lupus is often noted in children of color. The lesions in Fig. 9.2 were noted at birth in a Hispanic infant with progressive exacerbation over the first few weeks of life. Her raccoon eyes were erythematous and telangiectatic, as would be noted in children of lighter skin tones. In a recent series of Asian children from Bangkok with neonatal lupus, the leading findings in the skin were erythematous patches (91.7%), subacute lupus (50%), petechiae (41.7%), persistent cutis marmorata (16.7%) and discoid lesions (8.3%) [4] (Table 9.1).

Neonatal Lupus-CMTC-Like Clinical Appearance (Fig. 9.4)

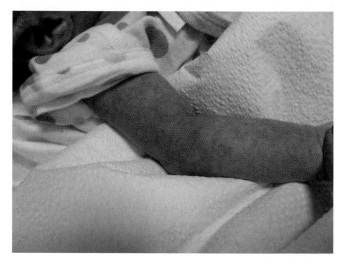

This newborn Hispanic infant appears to have cutis marmorata (Fig. 9.4); however she actually has neonatal lupus complicated by a positive anti-Ro antibody and platelet count reductions that required therapy with intravenous gammaglobulin. The skin findings resolved within a few weeks. CMTC is not often noted in children of type V or VI skin type. As a result, neonatal lupus should be considered in children of color when CMTC-like lesions are noted. These lesions resolved partially with swaddling, indicating they were not vascular malformations [5].

Neonatal Lupus-Sequelae (Figs. 9.5 and 9.6)

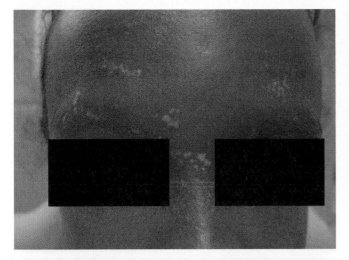

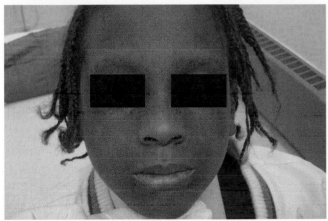

In children with darker skin tones, periorificial lesions are often bullous, heeling with atrophic scarring and pigmentary alterations ranging from early hypopigmentation as noted in the child in Fig. 9.5, to late hyperpigmentation as noted in the subsequent figure (Fig. 9.6). Hyperpigmentation is common sequelae of neonatal lupus, noted months to years after lesion clearance.

Systemic Lupus Erythematosus (Figs. 9.7–9.9)

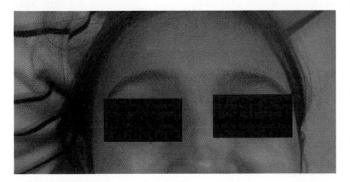

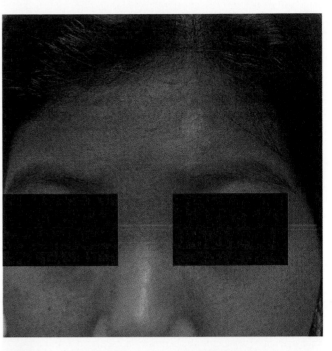

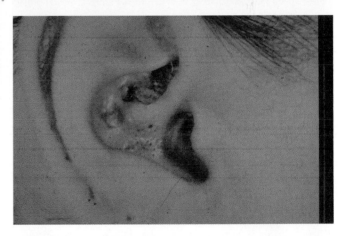

Systemic lupus erythematosus is a multi-system autoimmune disorder typified by production of antinuclear antibodies. The 7-year-old Caucasian female in Fig. 9.7 has systemic lupus erythematosus and a malar rash as a result of sun exposure. The malar rash is usually a mildly indurated erythema of the medial cheeks and nasal bridge, sparing the nasolabial fold. Lesions are most notable due to bright erythema in Caucasian children, with less prominence in Asian (Fig. 9.8) children and progressive obfuscation with progressive increases in cutaneous pigmentation.

The ACR criteria for the diagnosis of systemic lupus require 4 or more of 11 criteria to be met, the mucocutaneous criteria being malar rash, photosensitivity, discoid lupus (annular scaly plaques with scarring and atrophy) (Fig. 9.9) which is often noted in the ear as patulous pores and scarring, and oral ulcers (painless and asymptomatic). Other lupus lesions include subacute cutaneous lupus, in which annular indurated plaques are noted (Table 9.2).

Table 9.2 The ACR criteria for systemic lupus erythematosus

Malar rash
Discoid rashes
Photosensitivity
Oral ulcers
Arthritis (nonerosive, two or more joints)
Serositis (pleuritis or pericarditis)
Renal disorder (proteinuria or cellular casts)
Neurological (seizures or psychiatric)
Hematologic disorder
Immunologic abnormalities (Smith, dsDNA, false positive syphilis)
Antinuclear antibody (in the absence of drug-induced causation)

Poikiloderma (Figs. 9.10 and 9.11)

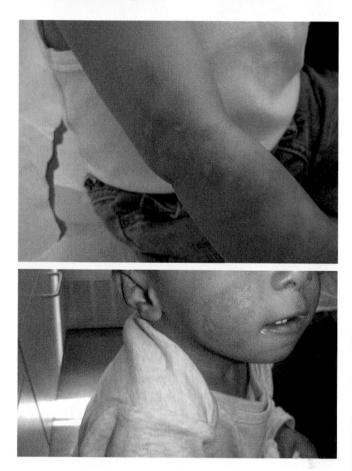

Poikiloderma is the combination of hyperpigmentation, hypopigmentation, and telangiectasias. This trio of findings is the main finding in poikiloderma congenitale (Figs. 9.10 and 9.11) (Rothmund Thomson Syndrome OMIM, 268400) an autosomal recessive disorder caused by a genetic defect of the REcQ4 gene and typified by poikiloderma, silvery hair, saddle nose deformity and potentially, tumors of the long bones.

Ephelides (Fig. 9.12)

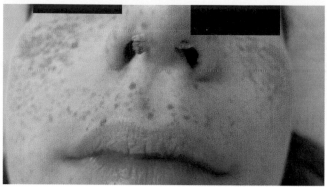

Ephelides or freckles (Fig. 9.17) are noted in light Caucasian children who have had sunburns. Freckles are a marker of DNA alteration from UV exposure. Individuals with ephelides require sun protection and careful monitoring. This child came in to be evaluated for wart therapy, without making mention of her ephelides. Few white individuals understand that freckles or ephelides are a marker of sun damage, as it is considered an attractive childhood skin feature. This lack of concern with ephelides is similar to the lack of concern people have with tanning.

Extensive Sun Damage in a Redhead (Fig. 9.13)

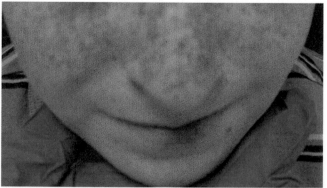

Not all children who develop phototoxic reactions are photosensitive. This redhead was worked up for ultraviolet light sensitivity, but had developed sun damage merely because he has Fitzpatrick phototype I skin and refused to use sun protection (Fig. 9.13).

Infantile Sunburn (Fig. 9.14)

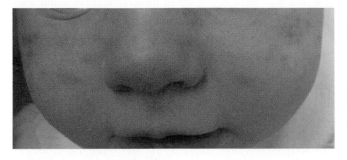

Infantile sunburns are exclusive to light-skinned children, whether Caucasian, light Asian, or light Hispanic children. Infantile sunburn is shown here in a red headed infant (Fig. 9.14) who got his sunburn through the car window. Early sunburn is very likely to increase melanoma risk [6].

Phytophotodermatitis (Figs. 9.15–9.17)

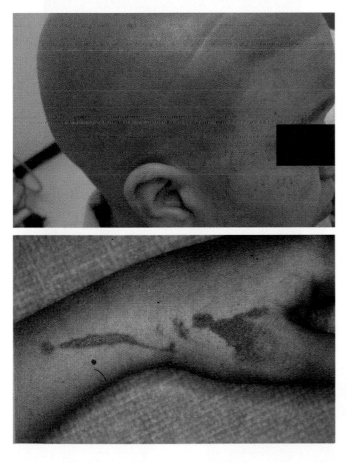

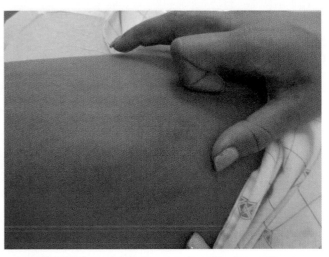

Table 9.3 Causes of phytophotodermatitis

Celery
Hogweed
Lemon
Lime
Mango
Parsley
Parsnip

Though photosensitivity is not common in children of color, cutaneous sensitizing agents can produce localized sunburn reactions, whether from iatrogenic causes as noted in the alopecia areata patient on topical psoralens and UVA for the scalp disease (Fig. 9.16) or from natural exposures, i.e., phytophotodermatitis (Fig. 9.17). In all children, these reactions are extremely dark and well defined. Although individuals of color are less likely to tan, iatrogenic exposure to psoralens, as noted in this African American female (Fig. 9.15), causes hyperpigmentation (i.e., tanning) when used for alopecia areata as noted in this patient (Table 9.3).

Morphea (Figs. 9.18–9.21)

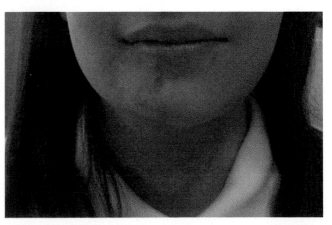

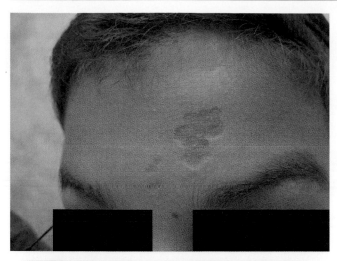

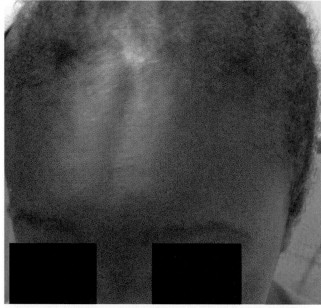

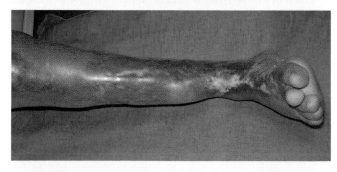

In Fig. 9.19, atrophic border edges are better demarcated due to the darker skin tone in this patient. In Fig. 9.20, broad depression of the underlying skin extends to the bony table and in a blaschkolinear path of atrophy and follicular loss, termed en coup de sabre. Black children will have notable hyperpigmentation associated with the inflammation, allowing for the recognition of disease extension. Linear morphea, which follows the lines of Blaschko, causes significant morbidity over joints by limiting mobility in terms of joint mobility (Fig. 9.21) and often requiring physical therapy. On the scalp, underlying brain inflammation can be seen with en coup de sabre, including migraines and seizure activity. MRI can be indicated. Methotrexate and oral corticosteroids can aid in achieving remission. Correction with surgery cannot be performed until years later, due to risk of traumatic disease reactivation. Hyaluronic acid fillers can be used to reduce the cosmetic defects.

Juvenile Dermatomyositis (Figs. 9.22–9.24)

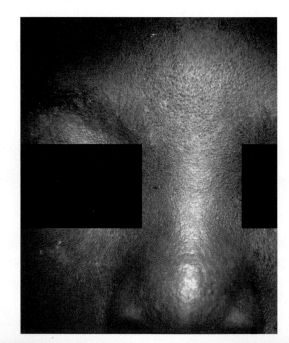

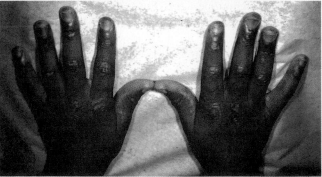

Morphea is a skin-limited form of inflammation causing bound down skin in a localized or linear fashion. More than half of cutaneous morphea patients have a positive antinuclear antibody test, the meaning of which is unknown, since cutaneous morphea is not considered a systemic autoimmunity.

In Fig. 9.18, one can note that morphea in a Caucasian child has a shadow effect that arises from atrophy and hyperpigmentation/violaceous (violet) hue of the depressed skin.

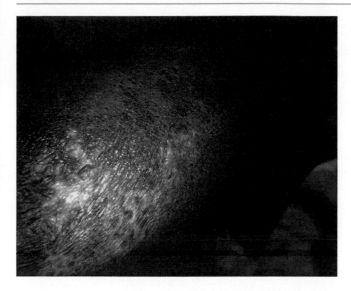

chest are often noted overlying the erythema of dermatomyositis in patients of dark skin tone. In contrast Caucasians often have violaceous erythema of sun-exposed areas [9].

Black children present with more dyspigmentation including hypopigmentation or hyperpigmentation (Figs. 9.23 and 9.24) overlying the lesions of the extremities [9]. This results in notable hyperpigmented plaques over the joints, sometimes obscuring the inflammation. This is true as well for the heliotrope sign (Fig. 9.22). In dark Hispanic (personal experience) and Black individuals, the heliotrope sign can appear as periocular hyperpigmentation [9]. Finally, nail capillaroscopy may be more difficult in darker children due to underlying pigment. Erythema of the gingival/the dental crown is generally not obscured by pigmentation and can be used as a consistent sign.

Juvenile dermatomyositis is an autoimmune/collagen vascular disease of childhood in which typical cutaneous manifestations are accompanied by muscular inflammation. Proximal muscle weakness with a positive Gower's sign and debilitating calcification of the musculature can be noted. When skin disease occurs in the absence of muscular inflammation, this is termed dermatomyositis sine myositis. Vasculopathy underlies the lesions of juvenile dermatomyositis. Diagnostic testing will reveal elevations in muscle enzymes and muscular changes on electromyography, MRI, ultrasound, and/or biopsy.

The typical skin manifestations of juvenile dermatomyositis include the heliotope rash (Fig. 9.22), which is a violaceous erythema and edema of the eyelids/periorbital skin, violaceous erythema/erythematous lichenoid papules/plaques over the joints of the knees, elbows and hands, and nail capillaroscopic abnormalities. In general, JDMS is far more common in Caucasian children (74%) than Black (14%), Asian (3%), and Hispanic (5%) children [7].

As with many conditions, detection of juvenile dermatomyositis can be affected by skin tone. First, the presence of pigment can obscure some of the violaceous quality of the vasculature in the skin as noted in the vague erythema and edema of the heliotrope sign in Fig. 9.22. Flagellate erythema of the back and zebra-like erythema of the extremities have been described as a feature in adult African patients and can be pruritic [8]. Hyperpigmentation of the face and V of the

References

1. Bhalla M, Garg G, Thami GP (2011) Photodistribution of rash in phenytoin-induced drug rash with eosinophilia and systemic symptoms. Clin Exp Dermatol 36(5):553–554
2. Mehta S, Lang B (1999) Long-term followup of naproxen-induced pseudoporphyria in juvenile rheumatoid arthritis. Arthritis Rheum 42(10):2252–2254
3. Borchers AT, Naguwa SM, Shoenfeld Y, Gershwin ME (2010) The geoepidemiology of systemic lupus erythematosus. Autoimmun Rev 9:A277–A287
4. Wisuthsarewong W, Soongswang J, Chantorn R (2011) Neonatal lupus erythematosus: clinical character, investigation, and outcome. Pediatr Dermatol 28:115–121
5. del Boz J, Serrano Mdel M, Gómez E, Vera A (2009) Neonatal lupus erythematosus and cutis marmorata telangiectatica congenita-like lesions. Int J Dermatol 48:1206–1208
6. Noonan FP, Recio JA, Takayama H, Duray P, Anver MR, Rush WL, De Fabo EC, Merlino G (2001) Neonatal sunburn and melanoma in mice. Nature 413:271–272
7. Pachman LM, Hayford JR, Hochberg MC, Pallansch MA, Chung A, Daugherty CD, Athreya BH, Bowyer SL, Fink CW, Gewanter HL, Jerath R, Lang BA, Szer IS, Sinacore J, Christensen ML, Dyer AR (1997) New-onset juvenile dermatomyositis: comparisons with a healthy cohort and children with juvenile rheumatoid arthritis. Arthritis Rheum 40:1526–1533
8. Diallo M, Fall AK, Diallo I, Diédhiou I, Ba PS, Diagne M, Ndiaye B, Ndiaye A, Niang A, Gning SB, Ba FK, Fall F, Mbaye PS (2010) Dermatomyositis and polymyositis: 21 cases in Senegal. Med Trop (Mars) 70:166–168
9. Dugan EM, Huber AM, Miller FW, Rider LG (2009) International Myositis Assessment and Clinical Studies Group. Photoessay of the cutaneous manifestations of the idiopathic inflammatory myopathies. Dermatol Online J 15:1

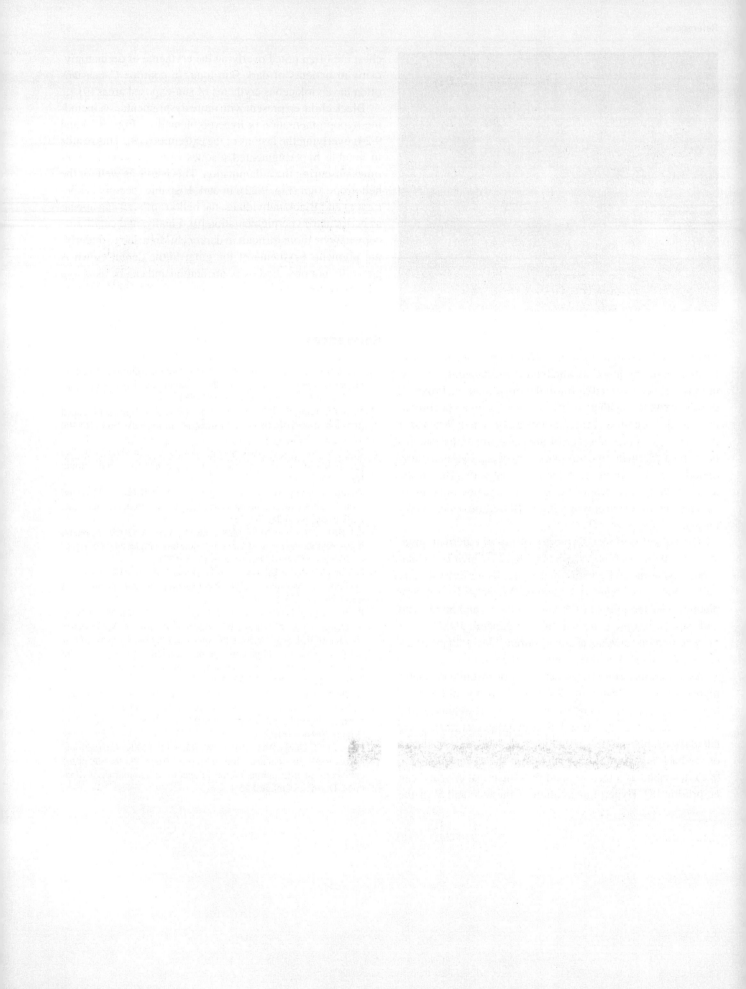

Lipoid Proteinosis (Figs. 10.1 and 10.2)

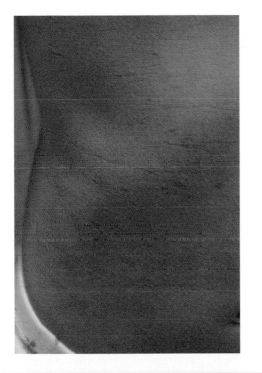

Lipoid proteinosis (Figs. 10.1 and 10.2) or Urbach–Wiethe disease (Hyalinosis Cutis et Mucosae) is caused by mutation of the ECM1 gene on chromosome 1q21.3. The disease is autosomal recessive with some increased prevalence in South Africa Afrikaner (0.07 prevalence) and in consanguineous Middle Eastern families. Thickening of the skin and mucosae is accompanied by beading along the eyelid margin and laryngeal infiltration/hoarseness. This Asian child has a hoarse voice and scarlike or poxlike lesions [1]. Anetodermic and atrophic scarring in my practice are most common in Asian children and consideration of lipoid proteinosis should be included in the differential of scarring.

Striae (Figs. 10.3–10.7)

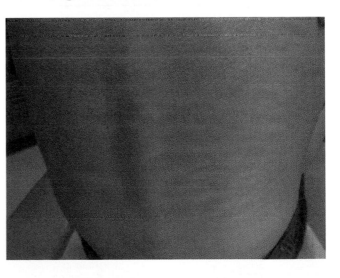

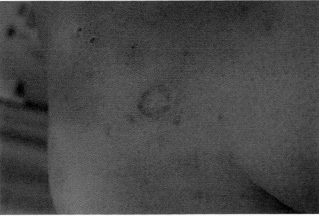

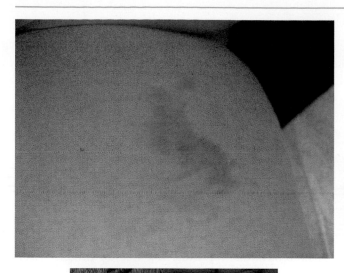

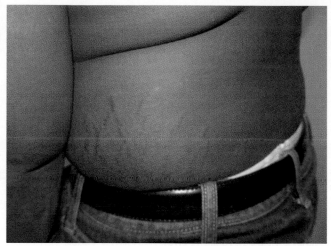

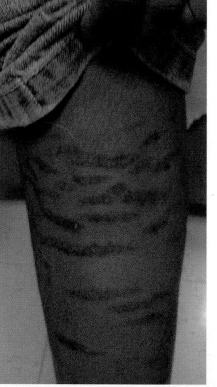

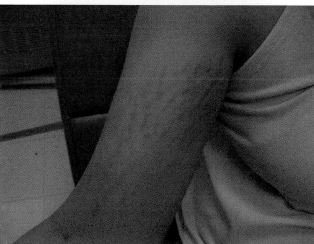

Striae distensae are thinned or atrophic areas of skin, often parallel to each other, occurring in 50–70% of teenage females. Striae are linear to fusiform, generally orienting perpendicular to the direction of growth in areas of rapid growth, such as the hips and upper thighs in girls and the knees in boys [2]. Coloration of striae has been described as white (Striae albae), reddish (Striae rubrae), bluish (Striae caeruleae) with corticosteroid therapy and blackish (Striae nigrae) in individuals of color.

In the Hispanic male in Fig. 10.3, horizontal striae over the back highlight a recent growth spurt. Notable hypopigmentation of the striae (Striae albae) demonstrates the long-term appearance of stretch marks in individuals of color after fading of erythema. In an individual with stigmata, such as pectus excavatum or carinatum, extensive striae from ages 10 to 18 years of age can be a sign of Marfan's disease. Cardiology, genetic, and ocular evaluations are required in suspected cases [3].

In the Caucasian preteen in Fig. 10.4, striae developed over the thighs due to use of corticosteroid agents topically. In my experience, application of corticosteroids is most likely to cause thinning in obese individuals and teenagers. In Caucasians, striae begin with erythematous (Striae rubrae) to violaceous (Striae Ceruleae) hue, amenable to pulsed dye laser. Unlike the darker patient of Fig. 10.5, the striae are erythematous without excess pigmentation.

Striae in Asian patients (Fig. 10.6), like Caucasian patients, demonstrate prominent erythema. In this Asian teenager, striae began after initiation of corticosteroids orally for systemic lupus erythematosus. She had a good reduction in lesional erythema and prominence with pulsed dye laser.

Striae in Black patients are dark as shown in Fig. 10.7 (Striae nigrae) progressing with time to hypopigmentation (Striae albae). On dermoscopy, Striae nigrae in individuals of color demonstrate a laddering melanization in rows perpendicular to the long axis of the striae, while Striae albae demonstrate an absence or disruption of the pigment network [4].

Judicious application of low to mid-potency corticosteroids, or choice of calcineurin inhibitors, is ideal for thin areas of skin such as the face and intertriginous regions to avoid striae development.

Granuloma Annulare (Figs. 10.8 and 10.9)

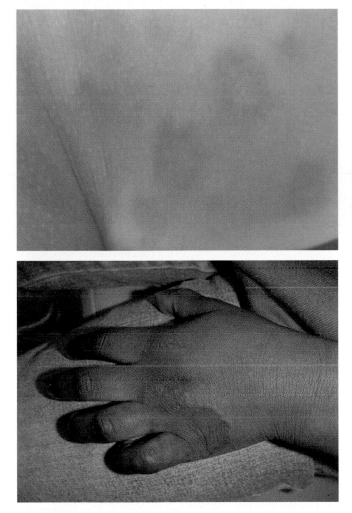

Granuloma annulare is an inflammatory dermal disorder, histologically typified by granulomatous inflammation and mucin deposition. Granuloma annulare can be triggered by environmental etiologies, such as bug bites. In adults and occasionally in teens, granuloma annulare can be associated with diabetes mellitus. Most reported granuloma annulare cases of childhood have been reported in Caucasian, Hispanic, or Asian children, however, there are no incidence studies that have been reported in children from a mixed population clinic comparing racial or ethnic incidence.

In childhood, average age is 8.6 years, with a male predominance. Lesions are typified by infiltrated plaques with beaded border, which consists of arcuate arrangement of firm papules (Fig. 10.8). Solitary lesions (54.7%), two lesions (16.6%), and 28.5% with three or more lesions. 92.8% of lesions resolve in 2 years [5]. Dermal nodules over the pretibial and forehead areas can be noted. These do not vary in appearance by race. Lesions

can last for a few years when untreated. Mid-potency topical corticosteroids, topical calcineurin inhibitors, and oral griseofulvin have been noted to be helpful in lesion clearance. Biopsy may be required in atypical cases.

Although, I cannot identify a citation that reviews this phenomenon, Granuloma Annulare in African American children demonstrate raised border of firm papules and central hyperpigmentation and hyperpigmentation on the inside of the border of beaded papules as shown in Fig. 10.9.

Atrophic Scar (Fig. 10.10)

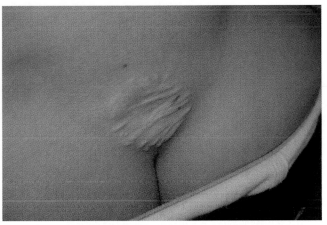

Atrophic scars (Fig. 10.10) appear hypopigmented with prominent vascularity in Caucasian children, as noted in this boy whose heavy activity level dehisced an excision site.

Urticaria (Fig. 10.11)

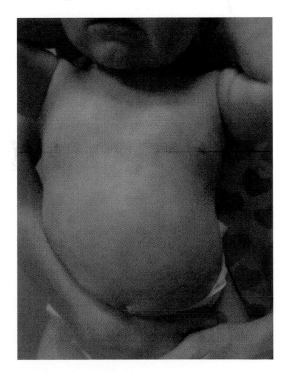

Table 10.1 Workup for chronic urticaria of childhood

Thyroid screen
Antinuclear antibody
Complete blood count
Complete metabolic profile
Urinalysis
Epstein Barr virus titers
Antistreptolysin antibodies
Hepatitis screen
IgE
C1, C2, C4 (C1 esterase inhibitor levels when angioedema predominates)
Ova and parasites (three times) for recent travel history
ESR picks up familial inflammasome-mediated cases (e.g., Muckle Wells)

Table 10.2 Therapy for urticaria

Antihistamines
Three levels
Fast acting (H1)
Diphenhydramine
Hydroxyzine
Chlorpheniramine
Long acting (H1)
Cetirizine
Loratidine/desloratidine
Fexofenadine
Long acting (non-H1) cimetidine, cyproheptadine, immunosuppressants
For people with inflammasome-mediated diseases newer agents that affect IL-1 production are available: antibodies to IL-1B (Canakinumab, Ilara®), IL-1 antagonist (Anakinra, Kineret®)
Epinephrine autoinjectors should be prescribed for angioedema or for documented severe allergies to seafood, peanuts, and bees
(<30 kg) 0.3 mL=0.15 mg epinephrine
(≥30 kg) 0.3 mL=0.3 mg epinephrine

Urticaria (Fig. 10.11) is a dermal edema of allergic origin caused usually by Type I, IgE-mediated allergic reaction to external agents such as foods, bee stings (Hymenoptera), medications, and infectious agents. Lesions are characterized by wheal and flare, i.e., blanching erythematous and indurated areas. The erythema of the flare of the urticaria is generally more notable in Caucasian and Asian children. Lesions in darker children can be obscured by background skin pigmentation (Tables 10.1 and 10.2).

In childhood, viral illnesses and food allergies are the leading causes [6], but *Streptococcal* infections can flare large urticarial episodes. Solar urticaria is also more common in Caucasian individuals [7]. Drug-induced urticaria caused by ACE inhibitors is more common in Black/Afro-Caribbeans [8].

Prolonged or chronic urticaria (>6 weeks) is usually caused by autoreactivity [9] caused by production of IgE anti-FCεR1 receptor antibodies. Other causes of chronic urticaria include hepatitis, autoimmune thyroid disease, and parasitic infections (e.g., *Strongyloides stercoralis*). Epinephrine autoinjectors should be prescribed for angioedema or for documented severe allergies to seafood, peanuts, and bees.

References

1. Nasir M, Latif A, Ajmal M, Qamar R, Naeem M, Hameed A (2011) Molecular analysis of lipoid proteinosis: identification of a novel nonsense mutation in the ECM1 gene in a Pakistani family. Diagn Pathol 6:69
2. Cho S, Park ES, Lee DH, Li K, Chung JH (2006) Clinical features and risk factors for striae distensae in Korean adolescents. J Eur Acad Dermatol Venereol 20:1108–1113
3. Faivre L, Masurel-Paulet A, Collod-Béroud G, Callewaert BL, Child AH, Stheneur C, Binquet C, Gautier E, Chevallier B, Huet F, Loeys BL, Arbustini E, Mayer K, Arslan-Kirchner M, Kiotsekoglou A, Comeglio P, Grasso M, Halliday DJ, Béroud C, Bonithon-Kopp C, Claustres M, Robinson PN, Adès L, De Backer J, Coucke P, Francke U, De Paepe A, Boileau C, Jondeau G (2009) Clinical and molecular study of 320 children with Marfan syndrome and related type I fibrillinopathies in a series of 1009 probands with pathogenic FBN1 mutations. Pediatrics 123:391–398
4. Piérard-Franchimont C, Hermanns JF, Hermanns-Lê T, Piérard GE (2005) Striae distensae in darker skin types: the influence of melanocyte mechanobiology. J Cosmet Dermatol 4(3):174–178
5. Martinón-Torres F, Martinón-Sánchez JM (1999) Martinón-Sánchez F localized granuloma annulare in children: a review of 42 cases. Eur J Pediatr 158(10):866
6. Konstantinou GN, Papadopoulos NG, Tavladaki T, Tsekoura T, Tsilimigaki A, Grattan CE (2011) Childhood acute urticaria in northern and southern Europe shows a similar epidemiological pattern and significant meteorological influences. Pediatr Allergy Immunol 22(1 pt 1):36–42
7. Kerr HA, Lim HW (2007) Photodermatoses in African Americans: a retrospective analysis of 135 patients over a 7-year period. J Am Acad Dermatol 57:638–643
8. Gibbs CR, Lip GY, Beevers DG (1999) Angioedema due to ACE inhibitors: increased risk in patients of African origin. Br J Clin Pharmacol 48(6):861–865
9. Sahiner UM, Civelek E, Tuncer A, Yavuz ST, Karabulut E, Sackesen C, Sekerel BE (2011) Chronic urticaria: etiology and natural course in children. Int Arch Allergy Immunol 156(2):224–230

Loose Anagen Syndrome (Fig. 11.1)

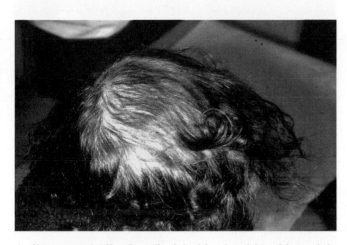

A disease typically described in blonde girls with straight hair, this illness manifests with difficulty growing long hair, easy removal of hairs, and nuchal textural alterations that cause the hairs to stand upward rather than lie flat. Easy removal of anagen hairs with gentle traction is noted, resulting in diffuse or patchy alopecia. Many girls outgrow this in puberty. The loose anagen hair bulb (Fig. 11.1) will have normal pigmentation and the so-called "rumpled socks" cuticle and misshapen hair bulbs [1]. Loose anagen hairs in an adult can be indicative of diffuse alopecia areata.

Most cases of loose anagen syndrome have been reported in blonde children. However, a recent case series of Egyptian children, Fitzpatrick skin types III–IV highlighted that the disease can be noted in children of color and even in children with wavy or curly hair. Loose anagen syndrome in a young African American girl is tinea capitis until proven otherwise, as the presence in Black children has never been reported [2].

In Caucasian female toddlers, poor hair growth is often noted, termed short anagen syndrome, typified by reduced anagen duration. Hair pull reveals a higher ratio of telogen to anagen hairs. Resolution with age is generally noted in puberty and adulthood. While hairs will be fine even into adulthood, these girls often develop more prolonged anagen phases and longer hair lengths in puberty.

Trichorrhexis Nodosa (Fig. 11.2)

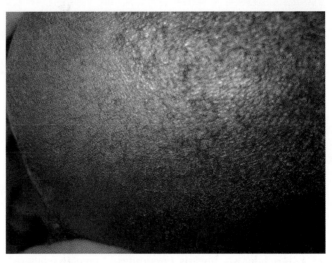

Trichorrhexis nodosa (Fig. 11.2) is a condition that can be inherited or acquired, in which hairs have fragile nodes that look like two broomsticks facing each other. Hair styling in African American girls such as blow-drying, ceramic flat iron usage, and aggressive combing seem to be exacerbants [3].

Trichorrhexis Invaginata (Figs. 11.3, 11.4)

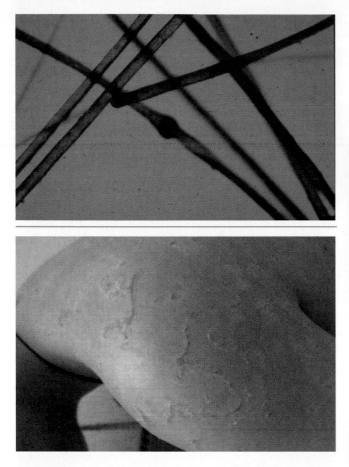

adolescents may improve growth of hair. In particular, diagnosis of monilethrix can be done using trichoscopy in vivo [5]. In children of color, the density of hair close to the scalp and background scalp pigmentation may obscure trichoscopy, necessitating taking hair clippings [6].

Traction Alopecia: Football-Shaped Alopecia (Figs. 11.5, 11.6)

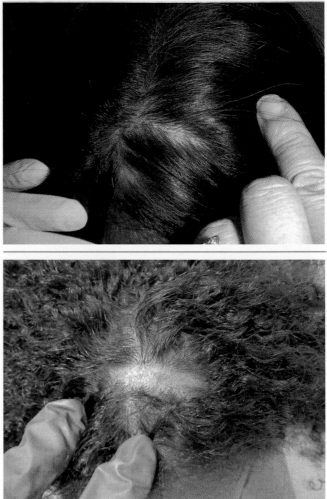

Trichorrhexis Invaginata or bamboo hairs (Fig. 11.3) are hairs with a ball and socket appearance and are noted in Netherton syndrome. In this picture, bamboo hairs are noted on microscopy. Dermoscopy (20–70×) in vivo over the lateral brow can be performed in Caucasian individuals to identify bamboo hairs. In individuals with dark pigmentation, higher magnification (70×, rather than 20×) and clipping of hairs for microscopy or in vitro dermoscopy against a white background can aid in visualization of shaft anomalies [4]. The clinical skin finding of Netherton syndrome as shown in Fig. 11.4, is ichthyosis linearis circumflexa, annular ichthyosis with double-edged scale. A clinical mimic can be seen when tinea corporis is found in children with congenital ichthyosis.

Monilethrix

Monilethrix is a genetic hair disorder caused by genetic alterations in hair cortex keratin genes and characterized by beading of the hair with intermittent constrictions. Hair fragility, occipital alopecia and difficulty growing hair will be noted, but improve with age. While most familial cohorts reported in the literature have been Caucasian, any race or ethnicity can be affected. Usage of topical minoxidil in

Alopecia areata is an autoimmune form of hair loss that has genetic rudiments in aberrant T and B cell activity and alterations in hair proteins. In girls of color, especially Hispanic girls with long, thick hair, who style their hair with tight ponytails, alopecia areata and traction alopecia will overlap in the central scalp in an ovoid or football-shaped pattern (Figs. 11.5 and 11.6), where the long-axis is parallel to the hairline. While these lesions will initially demonstrate swarm of bees on histology, in contrast to alopecia areata which resolves spontaneously in most children after 2 years, permanent alopecia may occur in these girls if high traction hair styles are not discontinued.

Traction Folliculitis (Fig. 11.7)

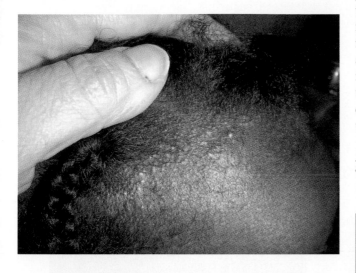

One of the early signs of hair follicle inflammation due to traction is folliculitis (Fig. 11.7). These cases typically present with follicular erythema, pustules and prominence along the hairline anteriorly, especially at the temples and result from tight ponytails, braids, and cornrows [7]. Prolonged traction folliculitis can result in alopecia, especially in chemically relaxed hair [8].

Traction Alopecia (Fig. 11.8)

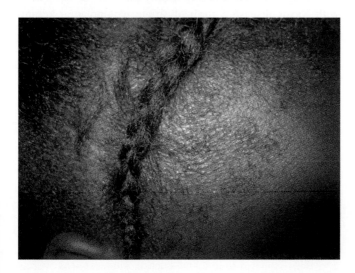

Traction alopecia is a form of hair loss that occurs in areas of high traction. Traction alopecia is especially common in Black girls across the frontal hairline. Prolonged traction, particularly in young girls whose hair has not achieved full thickness (usually under the age of 6 years) will result in permanent loss of the frontal hair; however, hair loss from traction can occur at any age. In teenage girls, hair loss from traction may be exacerbated by chemical damage from relaxers. If traction hair styles are discontinued soon after onset of hair loss, the hair may regrow; however, permanent loss is typical if high traction hair styles are continued. Traction alopecia of early childhood may be the root cause of Central Centrifugal Cicatricial Alopecia in adult women of color [9].

Trichoptilosis (Fig. 11.9)

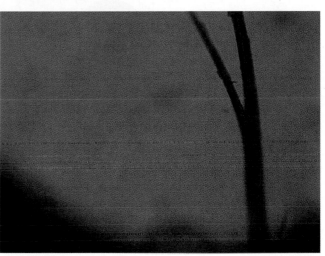

Trichoptilosis (Fig. 11.9), known in the vernacular as split ends, is a longitudinal splitting or fraying of the hair that can occur in any race or ethnicity. In Caucasian girls with long hair, split ends will be noted at the distal ends of the shafts as a marker of weakening of the cuticle with prolonged hair age. Exacerbation with over washing, chemical application including hair dyes and permanent therapies, excessive brushing and with blow-drying. A recent report of trichoptilosis from excessive hair gel usage highlights the susceptibility of the hair shaft in children of color to hair styling aids. In Black girls, the trichoptilosis may occur closer to the scalp as a result of hot combing and processing, or as a result of usage of ketoconazole or selenium sulfide shampoos [10].

Bubble hairs (bubbles or intra-shaft splitting) are also a style-induced damage that can also be noted in individuals who use hot combs, curling or straightening irons. As a result, it is quite common in teenage girls of color who use heat-related techniques for straightening the hair.

Hypertrichosis (Fig. 11.10)

Wooly Hair Nevus (Fig. 11.11)

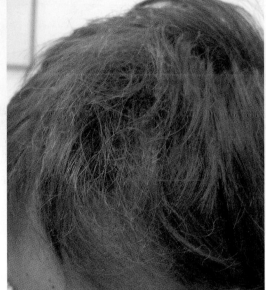

Hypertrichosis is a common finding in children from Middle Eastern backgrounds. Prominence of upper lip hair is noted more in Black than Caucasian adolescent girls 2 years after menarche, but can unlike generalized hypertrichosis noted in the Middle Eastern child, upper lip hair may improve slightly with age [11]. Typically there is a strong family history of hypertrichosis and a lack of early-virilization or premature adrenarche. In children with dark or course vellus hair of the body, especially in Hispanic and Middle Eastern children, notable hypertrichosis will be seen along the forehead, temples, neck, and upper back when high-potency corticosteroids are applied to the scalp for alopecia totalis (Fig. 11.10). Minoxidil topically on the scalp may cause the same side effect, and may further exacerbate this side effect when combined with high-potency topical corticosteroids.

Steroid-induced hypertrichosis resolves by 6 months after discontinuation of topical agents. A notable clinical feature in this child (who also has Down's syndrome) that was present prior to corticosteroid therapy is synophris, the merging of the brows over the glabellar region. Hair removal laser, waxing, electrolysis, and plucking are often used by hypertrichotic or hirsute patients for hair removal. Acne keloidalis nuchae and Pseudofolliculitis barbae may be precipitated by hair removal (these conditions are reviewed in Chap. 2).

While each individual has their own characteristic hair texture, thickness, and curvature, localized genetic or acquired alterations of hair growth patterns of the scalp can occur. In Caucasian children, these are often wooly hair nevi (Fig. 11.11), in which localized area of hair have an altered curvature and texture due to curved and elliptical hair shaft alterations [12]. Generalized wooly hair can be associated with Naxos disease a form of striate palmoplantar keratoderma with arrythmogenic right ventricular cardiomyopathy, which is relatively common in the Greek islands (1:1,000). A variant has been reported in India and Ecuador termed Carvajal syndrome [13]. Kinking or curling of the hair can be acquired locally after therapy of alopecia areata and generally with oral retinoid usage as well due to alterations of keratinization within the hair [14].

Straight Hair Nevus (Fig. 11.12)

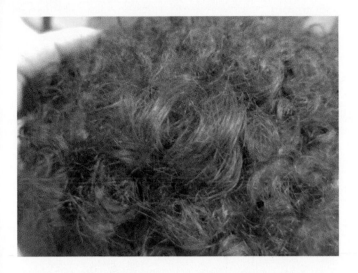

In this half Dominican and half African American boy, a straight hair nevus (Fig. 11.12) is noted among his curly hair. As a localized variant, hair straightening is more noticeable in a child of color with curly hair. In the absence of associated skin findings, this nevus represents a localized trichodysplasia with alteration in keratinogenesis of the cuticular cells [15].

Acquired alterations in hair color and texture have been described in alopecia areata patients after therapy. A case report of a 13-year-old African American boy who experienced hair straightening after localized topical corticosteroid application for alopecia areata has been described. In my practice, these changes often occur after hair regrowth following chemotherapy and when squaric acid immunotherapy is used for alopecia areata. The alterations in my patients generally resolve within a few years. HIV infection and malnutrition may also be causes of generalized, acquired hair straightening [16].

References

1. Dhurat RP, Deshpande DJ (2010) Loose anagen hair syndrome. Int J Trichol 2:96–100
2. Abdel-Raouf H, El-Din WH, Awad SS, Esmat A, Al-Khiat M, Abdel-Wahab H, Fakahani H, Al-Domyati M, El-Din Anber T, El-Tonsy MH (2009) Loose anagen hair syndrome in children of Upper Egypt. J Cosmet Dermatol 8:103–107
3. Martin AM, Sugathan P (2011) Localised acquired trichorrhexis nodosa of the scalp hair induced by a specific comb and combing habit – a report of three cases. Int J Trichol 3:34–37
4. Silverberg NB, Silverberg JI, Wong ML (2009) Trichoscopy using a handheld dermoscope: an in-office technique to diagnose genetic disease of the hair. Arch Dermatol 145:600–601
5. Liu CI, Hsu CH (2008) Rapid diagnosis of monilethrix using dermoscopy. Br J Dermatol 159:741–743
6. Silverberg NB, Silverberg JI, Wong ML (2009) Trichoscopy using a handheld dermoscope: an in-office technique to diagnose genetic disease of the hair. Arch Dermatol 145:600–601
7. Fox GN, Stausmire JM, Mehregan DR (2007) Traction folliculitis: an underreported entity. Cutis 79:26–30
8. Khumalo NP, Jessop S, Gumedze F, Ehrlich R (2007) Hairdressing is associated with scalp disease in African schoolchildren. Br J Dermatol 157:106–110
9. Shah SK, Alvarez MS, Hawit F, Alexis AF, Silverberg NB (2007) Selected topics in pediatric hair loss. Exp Rev Dermatol 2:795–804
10. Lee HW, Choi JH, Moon KC, Koh JK (2008) Trichoptilosis developing after first exposure to hair gels. Pediatr Dermatol 25:139–140
11. Lucky AW, Biro FM, Daniels SR, Cedars MI, Khoury PR, Morrison JA (2001) The prevalence of upper lip hair in black and white girls during puberty: a new standard. J Pediatr 138:134–136
12. Reda AM, Rogers RS 3rd, Peters MS (1990) Woolly hair nevus. J Am Acad Dermatol 22:377–380
13. Meera G, Prabhavathy D, Jayakumar S, Tharini G (2010) Naxos disease in two siblings. Int J Trichol 2:53–55
14. Graham RM, James MP, Ferguson DJ, Guerrier CW (1985) Acquired kinking of the hair associated with etretinate therapy. Clin Exp Dermatol 10:426–431
15. Downham TF 2nd, Chapel TA, Lupulescu AP (1976) Straight-hair nevus syndrome: a case report with scanning electron microscopic findings of hair morphology. Int J Dermatol 15:438–443
16. Valins W, Vega J, Amini S, Woolery-Lloyd H, Schachner L (2011) Alteration in hair texture following regrowth in alopecia areata: a case report. Arch Dermatol 147:1297–1299

Acquired Tumors of Childhood and Posttraumatic Events

Keloids (Figs. 12.1 and 12.2)

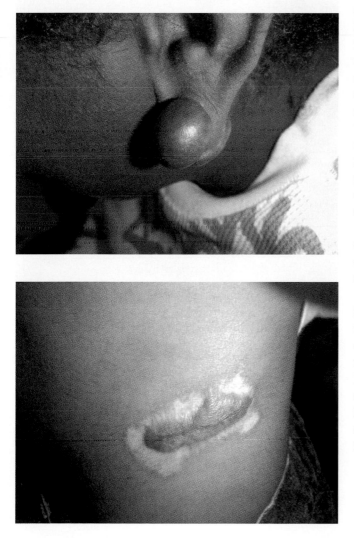

Keloids are benign fibroproliferative tumors that occur as excessive fibrous tissue response or exaggerated scars, forming after traumas such as surgery, piercings, and tattoos. While keloids usually form after puberty, occasionally keloids occur in young children with a familial tendency. Sites of keloids include earlobes (Fig. 12.1), central chest, upper arms, face/neck, and lower limbs. Linear (Fig. 12.2), bulbous and butterfly-shaped firm erythematous to flesh-colored lesions have been described [1]. Keloids are felt to be autosomal dominant with variable expression. Most familial cases are found in Blacks (up to 16% of Black individuals), but Caucasian and Asian families have been described [2]. Individuals of color are more prone to keloids, including Hispanics and Asians and keloids constitute one of the top ten diagnoses treated in a population of color [3].

Piercings are common practice in children of all colors and are currently perceived as socially acceptable. Infections, tooth chipping, bleeding, keloids, allergic reactions, and bruising are common side effects noted by teens with piercings [4].

Therapy is similar in all skin types, races and ethnicities, including intralesional kenalog injections, debulking, and intralesional interferon. Corticosteroid impregnated tapes can be tried in needle-phobic children with keloids. Radiation therapy is inadvisable postoperatively in young children. Infantile ear piercing in susceptible infants is the best form of earlobe keloid prevention, as keloids are rare in infancy; however, keloids do rarely occur in infants and a single case of prenatal keloid development due to fetal blood sampling has been described [5].

N.B. Silverberg, *Atlas of Pediatric Cutaneous Biodiversity: Comparative Dermatologic Atlas of Pediatric Skin of All Colors,*
DOI 10.1007/978-1-4614-3564-8_12, © Springer Science+Business Media, LLC 2012

Syringomas (Fig. 12.3)

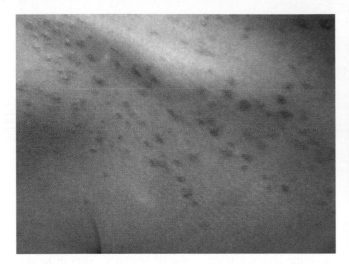

Syringomas are benign tumors of the eccrine gland that appear as small, translucent papules, usually in a periocular distribution. Asian women and Down syndrome patients are the grouping most affected, and these individuals will develop lesions beginning in early adolescence. Eruptive onset has been described in children of color ages 4–8 years over the chest, axillae, abdomen, and proximal extremities [6].

In Asian patients, the lesions are yellow-pink to flesh-colored. Lesions of syringomas are more pigmented to orange in Hispanic patients due to background pigmentation. Electrocautery, cryotherapy and pulsed dye laser may both aid in lesion size reduction. Pre- or post-treatment hydroquinoine therapy may help reduce dyspigmentation.

Syringomas can be familial as in the patient depicted in Fig. 12.3. Lesions are more often on the neck and upper chest in Black patients demonstrating dark brown, hyperpigmentation to violaceous appearance. Therapy in individuals of color may be complicated by hyperpigmentation postprocedurally, keloid formation especially over the sternal area and hypopigmentation if treated with invasive procedures. For this reason, small test areas should be used prior to therapy of larger surface areas in this grouping.

Dermatofibromas (Figs. 12.4 and 12.5)

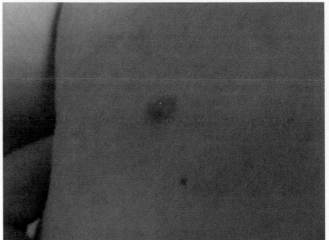

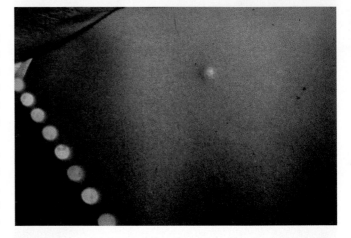

Dermatofibromas (benign fibrous histiocytoma) are localized firm lesions that develop, on the legs or less frequently the arms. These lesions form in response to injuries, such as insect bites. Women are more likely to develop dermatofibromas. In Caucasians, the lesions run from flesh-colored nodules to medium brown (Fig. 12.4). In individuals of color, dermatofibromas can be very dark (Fig. 12.5), but dermoscopy will often demonstrate a central white scarlike patch and a thin rim of a fine pigment network. Multiple lesions can be seen in individuals with systemic lupus erythematosus, which is especially common in women of color, especially African American women.

Juvenile Xanthogranuloma (Figs. 12.6 and 12.7)

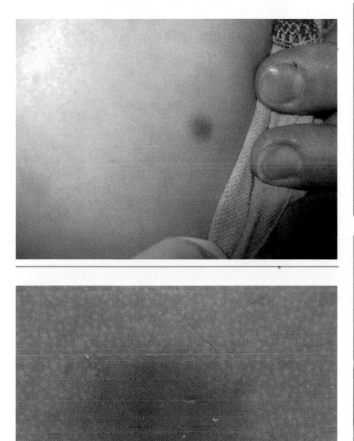

Mastocytoma (Figs. 12.8–12.10)

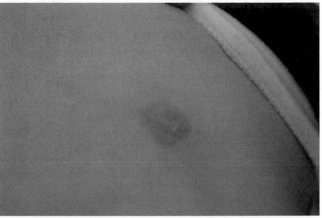

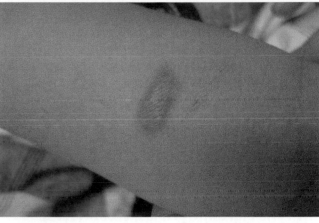

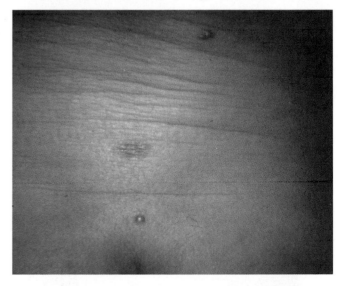

Juvenile xanthogranuloma is a benign tumor of infancy and early childhood. Solitary yellow-red lesions are common and will resolve with age. Yellow-orange coloration (Fig. 12.6) with smaller areas of lighter globules is noted on dermoscopy. Multiple lesions warrant a search for cafe au laits; when a comorbid diagnosis of neurofibromatosis type 1 is supported by physical examination, screening for CML has to be performed. Multiple lesions in the absence of cafe au lait macules warrant ophthalmology examination and close follow-up.

In children of color, the yellow-orange coloration of the JXG lesion is less notable, with lesions being tanner to brown. As a result of the firmness and coloration, larger JXG lesions in African American children can resemble hypertrophic scars or keloids [7]. Dermoscopy shows a fine reticular network in the orange yellow background (Fig. 12.7), even in this photo from the leg of an African American infant.

Cutaneous mastocytosis can be divided into five types in childhood, including cutaneous mastocytosis, indolent systemic mastocytosis, systemic mastocytosis with associated clonal hematologic illness of an origin other than the mast cell line, aggressive systemic mastocytosis, and mast cell leukemia. For the purpose of this book, I will review the clinical features of the cutaneous type. However, when systemic disease is suspected skin biopsy, complete blood counts with peripheral smears, abdominal ultrasound, tryptase levels, and bone marrow biopsies may play a role in determining disease extent [8].

A mastocytoma is a nevoid accumulation of mast cells in the skin. Mastocytomas fade with age and are often resolved by adulthood. Solitary lesions are generally tan to light brown, becoming pink with pressure. In darker children, lesions may be darker brown, but are rarely more than a shade or two darker than the background skin. Mastocytomas demonstrate urtication with exposure to mast cell degranulators (e.g., polymyxin B, alcohol, strawberries, aspirin), or with pressure-termed the Darier's sign. Urtication frequency, i.e., lesion lability appears to wane with time, prior to lesion clearance. In my practice, the vast majority of children with mastocytomas are either Caucasian, Asian or Hispanic, however, I cannot identify head-to-head comparative data in the literature. A very frequent clinical scenario is that urtication was treated by a parent with polymyxin B, resulting in blistering of the lesion.

Figures 12.8 and 12.9 demonstrate a mastocytoma in a Caucasian child; Fig. 12.9 shows Darier's sign, i.e., urtication with pressure. Figure 12.10 demonstrates a mastocytoma in a darker skinned child with darker coloration; however, urtication should still be observable with pressure despite coloration.

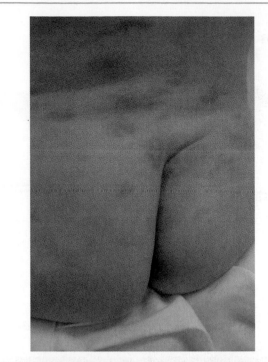

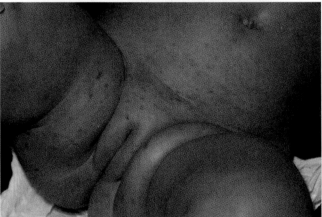

Urticaria Pigmentosa (Figs. 12.11–12.13)

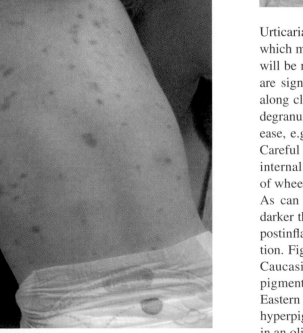

Urticaria pigmentosa is a form of cutaneous mastocytosis in which multiple lesions of the torso and proximal extremities will be noted. These lesions, especially in children of color, are significantly darker than the natural skin tone and fall along cleavage lines. Care must be taken to avoid mast cell degranulators due to risk of associated internal mast cell disease, e.g., lungs (wheezing) and gastrointestinal (diarrhea). Careful history and counseling regarding observation for internal findings is required including review of episodes of wheezing, flushing and abdominal cramps, and diarrhea. As can be noted in these figures, lesions are significantly darker than the normal skin tone. This may be as a result of postinflammatory changes due to frequent and intense urtication. Figure 12.11 demonstrates urticaria pigmentosum in a Caucasian child and Fig. 12.12 demonstrates urticaria pigmentosum with frictional urtication. The child of Middle Eastern descent in Fig. 12.13 demonstrates the depth of hyperpigmentation noted overlying urticaria pigmentosum in an olive skin tone child.

Diffuse Mastocytosis (Fig. 12.14)

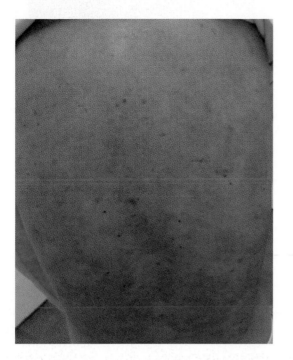

Diffuse mastocytosis (Fig. 12.14) is a cutaneous form in which mast cells accumulate broadly. In this Asian girl, broad areas of hyperpigmentation are noted. In Caucasian, Asian and light Hispanic patients, diffuse mastocytosis can give a dirty appearance to the skin. Hyperpigmentation can be lightened, as was done in this child, by initiation of daily antihistamines (in this case ranitidine) and a bleaching agent (hydroquinone 4%) concurrently.

References

1. Bayat A, Arscott G, Ollier WE, Ferguson MW, Mc Grouther DA (2004) Description of site-specific morphology of keloid phenotypes in an Afrocaribbean population. Br J Plast Surg 57: 122–133
2. Marneros AG, Norris JE, Olsen BR, Reichenberger E (2001) Clinical genetics of familial keloids. Arch Dermatol 137: 1429–1434
3. Child FJ, Fuller LC, Higgins EM, Du Vivier AW (1999) A study of the spectrum of skin disease occurring in a black population in south-east London. Br J Dermatol 141:512–517
4. Gold MA, Schorzman CM, Murray PJ, Downs J, Tolentino G (2005) Body piercing practices and attitudes among urban adolescents. J Adolesc Health 36:352.e17–e24
5. Birkhamshaw E, Gupta S (2011) An unusual complication of foetal blood sampling. Arch Dis Child 96:1065
6. Sacoor MF, Medley P (2004) Eruptive syringoma in four Black South African children. Clin Exp Dermatol 29(6):686–687
7. Ogawa R, Akaishi S, Hyakusoku H (2009) Differential and exclusive diagnosis of diseases that resemble keloids and hypertrophic scars. Ann Plast Surg 62:660–664
8. Heide R, Beishuizen A, De Groot H, Den Hollander JC, Van Doormaal JJ, De Monchy JG, Pasmans SG, Van Gysel D, Oranje AP (2008) Dutch National Mastocytosis Work Group. Mastocytosis in children: a protocol for management. Pediatr Dermatol 25: 493–500

Common Warts (Figs. 13.1, 13.2)

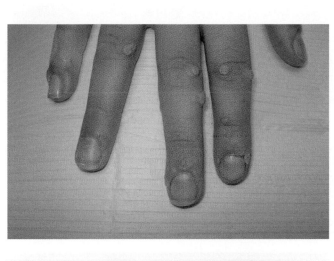

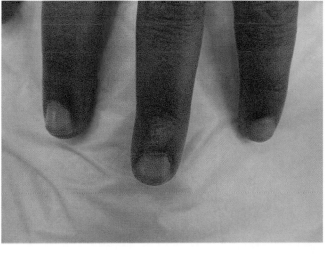

Common warts affect 20% of children and are generally caused by HPV 1 or 2. In my experience, lesions in Caucasians are flesh-colored to slightly hyperpigmented verrucous papules and plaques which are distinguished by lack of normal dermatoglyphics (Fig. 13.1). Unlike conditions like picker's nodules or lichen simplex chronicus, the hyperkeratotic skin

of common warts appears either flesh-colored or relatively hypopigmented even in patients of color, compared to the normal surrounding skin (Fig. 13.2). Rare patients will have pigmented warts with specific HPV types. These pigmented warts are darker in all patients.

Flat Warts (Figs. 13.3, 13.4)

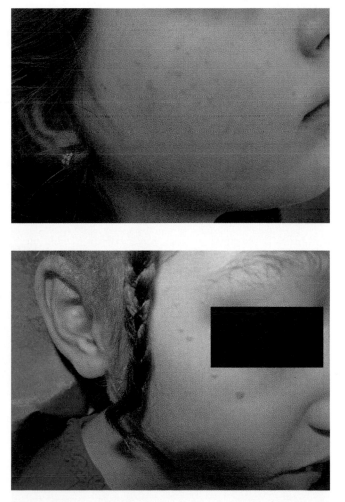

N.B. Silverberg, *Atlas of Pediatric Cutaneous Biodiversity: Comparative Dermatologic Atlas of Pediatric Skin of All Colors*,
DOI 10.1007/978-1-4614-3564-8_13, © Springer Science+Business Media, LLC 2012

Flat warts are caused by HPV 3 or 10 and in immunocompromised individuals, HPV 5 or 8. In all patients flat warts can range from hypopigmented to hyperpigmented flat-topped papules. In the Caucasian (Fig. 13.3) and Hispanic patient (Fig. 13.4) flat warts are flesh-colored to relatively tan 1–3 mm papules with abnormal dermatoglyphics. Epidermodysplasia verruciformis type lesions typify the broad range of pigmentation that can be seen in flat warts. In African patients epidermodysplasia verruciformis lesions can be flat and hypopigmented mimicking tinea versicolor or flat and hyperpigmented, mimicking tinea versicolor, porokeratosis (see Chap. 7) or lichen planus [1].

Linear distribution of flat warts may be noted when trauma, such as shaving, spread the lesions in a linear fashion. Treatments include peeling agents (e.g., tretinoin or glycolic acid), destructive agents (e.g., liquid nitrogen), and immunotherapies (e.g., imiquimod), but should be done cautiously in children of color, due to risk of pigmentary disturbance. Localized erythema and eczematous changes may be noted with the latter treatment [2].

Tinea Versicolor (Figs. 13.5, 13.6, 13.7, 13.8, 13.9)

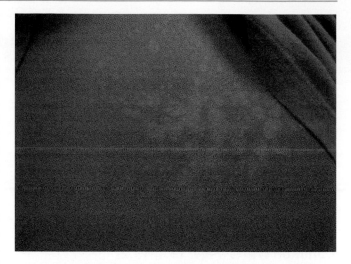

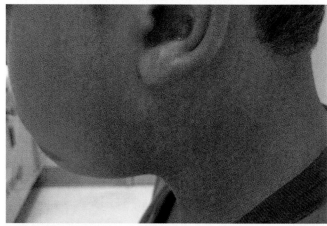

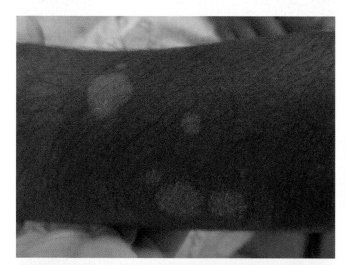

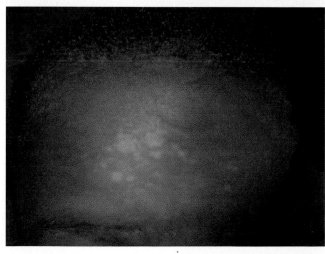

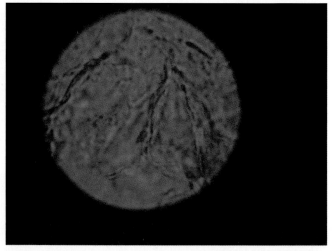

Tinea versicolor (pityriasis versicolor) is not a form of tinea, but rather, is caused by yeast overgrowth of the *Malassezia* species in the keratinized skin. In Caucasians, fine tan thin plaques are noted over the skin of the neck and trunk or upper extremities (Fig. 13.5). Tinea Versicolor usually occurs in post-pubertal individuals (Fig. 13.6). However, petalloid seborrheic dermatitis of the infant is essentially tinea versicolor. Lesions are generally guttate thin plaques over the face and upper trunk. In Hispanic infants, lesions are hyperpigmented, while African American infants will have hypopigmented lesions. Pityriasis versicolor is amongst the top conditions seen in a dermatology clinic in individuals of color [3]. Treatments include selenium sulfide lotion, topical azole antifungals, and oral azole antifungals.

Tinea Versicolor in Teenagers of Color (Figs. 13.7, 13.8)

Tinea versicolor (Figs. 13.7, 13.8) manifests with either hypopigmented or hyperpigmented plaques. Post-inflammatory pigmentary alterations are common and bothersome in individuals of color. Dyschromia is on the top five list of diseases for which black individuals seek skin care [3,4]. Black and Hispanic patients are more likely to be affected cosmetically than Caucasian individuals and males more so than females [5]. Immunosuppression may exacerbate disease.

In limited cases, treatments include selenium sulfide or azole antifungals, however, tinea versicolor often causes vague, broad areas of pigmentary alterations in children. As a result, short courses of oral azole antifungals may be needed to address overgrowth in these patients. In this patient the potassium hydroxide preparation corroborated the diagnosis (Fig. 13.9).

Tinea Capitis (Figs. 13.10, 13.11, 13.12, 13.13, 13.14, 13.15)

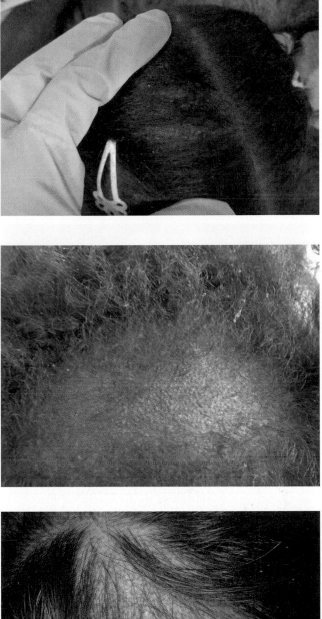

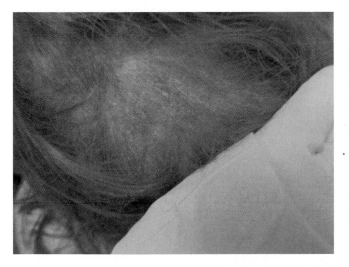

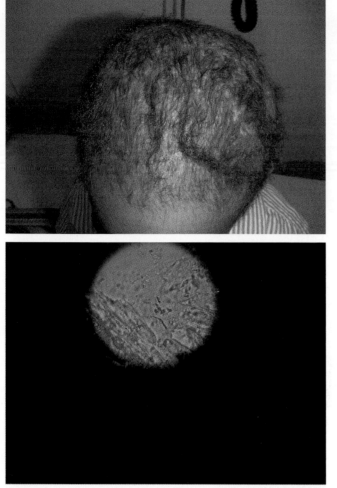

Table 13.1 Infections: the effect of race

Infections more common in caucasians
Lice
Infections more visible in caucasians
Scarlet fever
Viral exanthemata
Infections more common in black or hispanic children
Confluent and reticulated papillomatosis
Tinea capitis
Infections more visible in individuals of color
Progressive macular hypomelanosis
Tinea versicolor

Table 13.2 Treatment of tinea capitis

Household practice alterations/reduction of spread or reinfection through fomites	Avoid sharing hats, combs, brushes, pillowcases
	Wash hats, combs, brushes, pillowcases once a week in a hot water rinse to remove fungal fomites
	Selenium sulfide 1% shampoo for household members when washing [16]
	Conditioners to be used for index case and family members [17]
Shampoos and conditioners	Selenium sulfide 1% shampoo
	Ciclopirox 1% shampoo or
	2% ketoconazole shampoo twice-weekly as adjunctive therapy to aid in reducing infectivity and induce mycological cure [18,19]
Oral Antifungals (6 weeks minimum in most cases) – FDA-approved medications (dosages may vary from original monograph)	Griseofulvin 20–25 mg/kg/day of micronized suspension [20]
	Griseofulvin 10–12 mg/kg/day of ultramicronized tablets[1]
	Terbinafine sprinkles <25 kg 125 mg/day 25-35 kg 187.5 mg/day >35 kg 250 mg/day
Non-FDA-approved treatments for tinea capitis	Fluconazole 6 mg/kg/d 3–6 weeks
	Itraconazole 100 mg capsule daily in food for 4 weeks

Tinea capitis is a worldwide scalp dermatophyte infection of children of all colors; however, prevalence in Black children is 3–4 times that of Caucasian children (Table 13.1) [6]. The most common type is the seborrheic type (Figs. 13.10, 13.11), mimicking seborrheic dermatitis. Background carriage and infection in adults of color and siblings in the same household is higher in households of affected children and of individuals of color. As a direct result, the highest suspicion should be held that children of color with scalp hyperkeratosis ages 3–10 years have tinea capitis until proven otherwise. Infection with dermatophytes is even more likely when a child has both scalp hyperkeratosis and alopecia and/or cervical adenopathy [7]. Caucasian children and children 2 years and under or teenagers, respectively, are more likely to have atopic dermatitis and/or seborrheic dermatitis as the cause of fine scaling of the scalp, however, fungal culture should be performed when disease is unresponsive to standard therapy [8].

Black dot tinea (Fig. 13.12) is the second most common type of tinea capitis, so named because most children with infection have dark brown (black) hairs. Caucasian children with tinea capitis would have brown dot (Fig. 13.13) or yellow dots, which would be more difficult to note, but are corollaries in individuals of lighter hair color. Oral antifungals are always needed for 4–6 weeks or greater to resolve tinea capitis due to the presence of tinea inside the hairs at an area that would be too deep for a topical agent to penetrate (Table 13.2).

One of the confirmatory signs of tinea capitis is dermoscopy demonstrating tiny corkscrew hairs at the tips of black dot follicles on the scalp. These are distinctive from alopecia areata type tapered hairs (exclamation point) and are specific to children who are Black. Another less specific sign is the presence of tiny hair fragments on the q-tip when fungal cultures are taken. These hairs break because the leading cause of tinea capitis is an endothrix infection, weakening the shaft. In the United States, most cases are caused by *Trichophyton Tonsurans*.

Kerions (Fig. 13.14) are an inflammatory forms of tinea capitis including inflammation, pustules, and thickened boggy plaques of alopecia. Most kerions are associated with cervical lymphadenopathy. Swift initiation of antifungal therapy with griseofulvin (the gold standard) or some alternative agent (terbinafine, fluconazole, itraconazole) can eradicate the kerion. However, if bogginess and inflammation aren't corrected rapidly, permanent alopecia can be seen. In my experience, short courses (5–7 days) of oral corticosteroid therapy (0.5–1 mg/kg/day) may release hairs from the intense inflammation more rapidly; however, many cases of kerion resolve adequately without the addition of corticosteroids. Upon initiation of oral antifungals, patients with inflammatory tinea capitis may develop an Id reaction, a generalized hypersensitivity response. Judicious topical or oral corticosteroid therapy can help patients through this hurdle so that they may continue oral antifungal therapy.

In the African American child in Fig. 13.14, kerion can be quite violaceous. Examination of the scalp using a Wood's lamp to rule out fluorescing zoophilic and geophilic dermatophyte species (e.g., *Microsporum canis*, *Microsporum Audoini*) is required, but most kerions are caused by *Trichophyton tonsurans* in the United States. Fungal stains (Fig. 13.15) can help identify hyphae in fractured hairs in the standard endothrix of *Trichophyton Tonsurans*. Tinea capitis may have long-term sequelae. Adult African American women are more likely to develop central hair loss in adulthood, and tinea capitis earlier in life is a risk factor for this alopecia [9].

mulate on the hair shaft and demonstrate collections of spores on KOH examination. Disease has recently been reported in Hispanic/Latino and Middle Eastern girls with long hair and may be regionally more common, especially in Central and South America. While shaving the scalp was required in the past, it appears that usage of oral antifungals in the azole family paired with prolonged antifungal shampoos may allow individuals to clear scalp carriage and infection [10].

Molluscum Contagiosum (Figs. 13.17, 13.18, 13.19, 13.20)

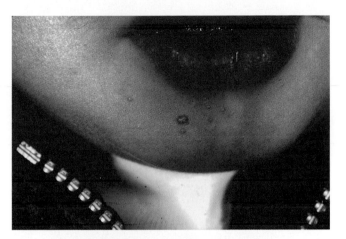

White Piedra (Fig. 13.16)

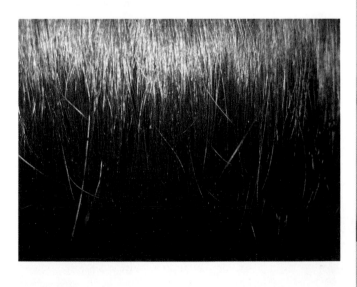

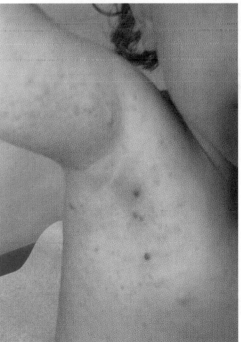

In the mimics of tinea capitis is white piedra (Fig. 13.16) a yeast infection of the scalp and hair with *Trichosporon* species. White concretions, which are not easily removed, accu-

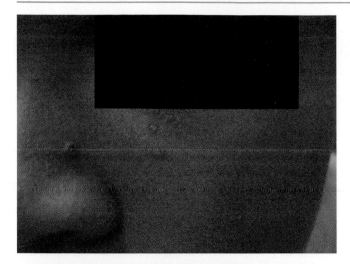

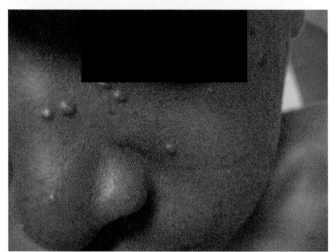

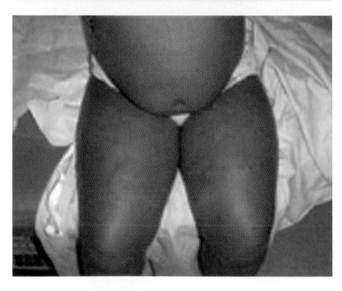

because lesions are tan or flesh-colored and have a small size (Fig. 13.17). There is a difficulty visualizing the central punctum in lesions under 2 mm in size.

Molluscum contagiosum virus affects all races and ethnicities and is associated with dermatitis in a third of children manifesting as erythema, eczematous lesions, and pruritus, obscuring the visualization of lesions (Fig. 13.18). Lesions in children of color may be flesh-colored to hypopigmented (Figs. 13.19 and 13.20). As follicular dermatitis is more common in children of color, follicular prominence and eczematous changes with hypopigmentation are often noted in Hispanic or Black children with molluscum infections.

In the African American child in Fig. 13.21, we note an eczematous dermatitis with a 2–3 cm radius around molluscum lesions, creating the appearance of target lesions of erythema multiforme. Therapy of dermatitis associated with molluscum unmasks lesions, allowing therapy of the underlying molluscum.

Confluent and Reticulated Papillomatosis of Gougerot and Carteaud (Figs. 13.22, 13.23)

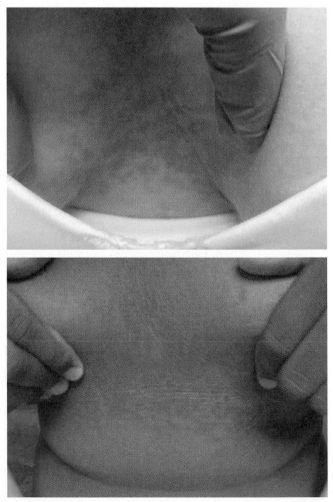

Molluscum contagiosum are caused by infection with the benign pox virus Molluscum Contagiosum Virus, of which there are four variants. Type 1 is the leading cause of pediatric infection. Molluscum contagiosum infections are often mistaken for milia cysts in younger Caucasian children

CARP is an infection with a species of bacteria termed *Dietzia papillomatosis* which causes this infection. [11] Velvety hyperpigmentation that is centrally confluent (in women this means confluence in the intermammary region) and reticulated on the underside of the breast and abdomen. Movement up the neck may overlap with acanthosis nigricans, as this infection seems more common in obese individuals. As can be noted here, Caucasian children will have tan plaques, but the morphology is the same in all skin tones (Fig. 13.22).

CARP is more noticeable in African American children due to dark discoloration (Fig. 13.23). Usage of oral minocycline 100 mg twice-daily will aid in clearance. Alternatives include mupirocin, isotretinoin, and calcipotriene. Due to the thickening of the skin, superimposed dirt or retention hyperkeratosis is not uncommon in overlying CARP (See Figs. 4.18, 4.19, 4.20) [12].

Tinea Pedis (Fig. 13.24)

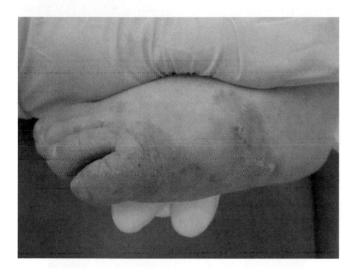

Tinea pedis is a common dermatophyte infection of the feet manifesting with hyperkeratosis of the soles and interdigital hyperkeratosis and maceration. Lesions may be more erythematous in Caucasian children, as seen in Fig. 13.24. Acquisition occurs from household contacts or gym/school or pool exposures. Walking barefoot, hyperhidrosis, and family history seem to increase the risk of infection. White cotton socks, cycling shoes to allow for full drying, application of azole or allylamine antifungals, and usage of sandals in high-exposure sites may aid in clearance of tinea pedis.

Bedbugs (Figs. 13.25, 13.26, 13.27)

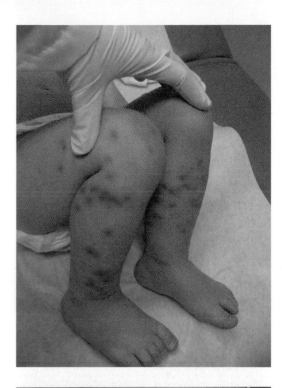

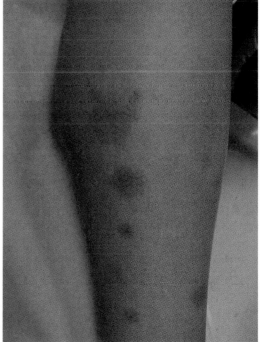

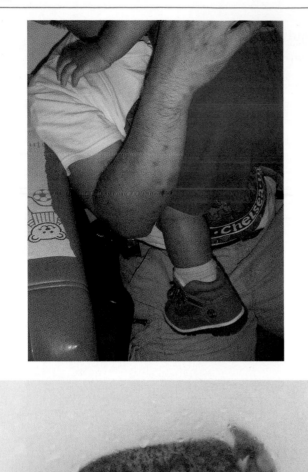

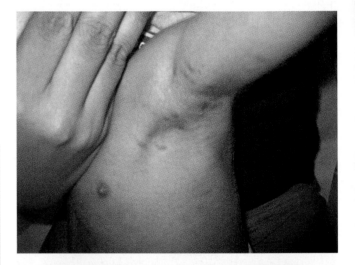

deeply violaceous bites due to bedbugs. Punctae may be somewhat obscured by pigment and magnification can aid in visualization of the same. Lesions in darker patients appear less violaceous because the background pigmentation obscures some of the erythema.

Dermoscopy can help identify bedbug samples (Fig. 13.28) brought in by patients as shown in the sample picture. This bug could crawl 1 foot per minute, so it is essential to keep specimens in well-sealed bags!!!

Scabies (Figs. 13.28–13.33)

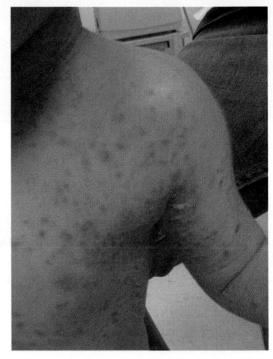

Bedbugs (Cimex lectularis) are small bugs that are frequently noted nowadays in cities around the United States. Bedbugs are equal opportunity biters, attacking children of all races and ethnicities after dark by living in mattresses and floorboards. Extermination is required to eradicate the infestation. Bites are often clustered with prominent punctae in Caucasian individuals (Fig. 13.25). Like all papular urticaria, the lesions are erythematous, but more intensely so than a mosquito bite and usually size lesions/reactions.

In the Asian family in Fig. 13.26, one can note deeply violaceous bites clustered on exposed regions in both a father and son. The Hispanic adolescent in Fig. 13.27 has

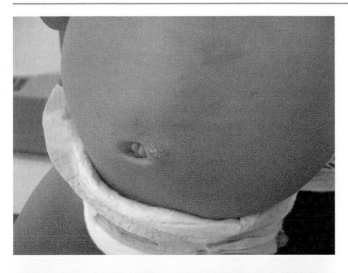

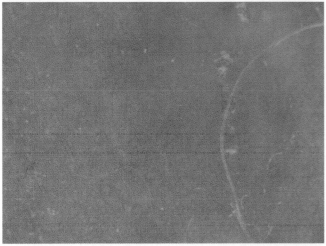

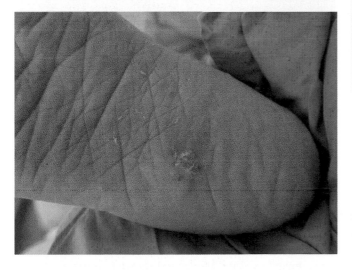

Scabies is a disease affecting all races and ethnicities. It is an infestation with the mite *Sarcoptes scabeii*. Treatment is usually permethrin 5% cream to the index and contacts twice (therapy overnight and 1 week apart) with careful cleaning of bedding and clothing, but infants require facial and scalp therapy. Infants and pregnant women can be treated with 6% precipitated sulfur. In the children in Figs. 13.29 and 13.30, we see the violaceous nodules of the axillae, the hallmark of infantile cases. Nodules can also be seen at the waistline and on the genitalia (Fig. 13.31). Dermoscopy of lesions can demonstrate tracts or burrows (Fig. 13.32). Nodules may be less prominently erythematous in children of color, but the risk of developing the sequela of Infantile Acropustulosis may be higher in Black and Hispanic infant males. The final picture (Fig. 13.33) demonstrates plantar lesions in a Black male infant, a lesion type not seen in individuals over the age of 2 years and possibly the rudiment of infantile acropustulosis.

Cutaneous Larva Migrans (Fig. 13.34)

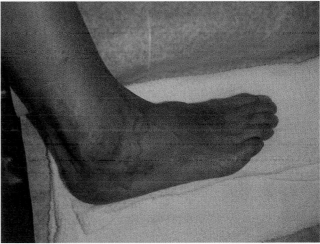

Patients acquire cutaneous larva migrans (Fig. 13.34) by walking or sitting barefoot on the beach where cats who were shedding the third stage of the nematode *Ancylostoma braziliensis* or *Ancylostoma duodenale*. Tropical environments are usual; therefore, worldwide the cases are most likely to be reported in travelers and individuals of color, especially Hispanic or Latino individuals. Treatment with topical thiabendazole or oral albendazole or ivermectin can aid in clearance [13].

Myiasis (Figs. 13.35, 13.36, 13.37)

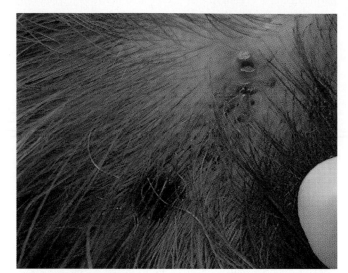

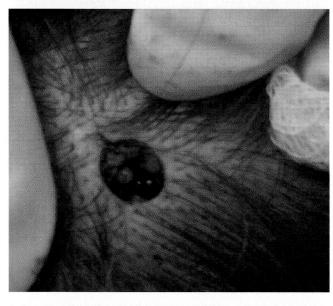

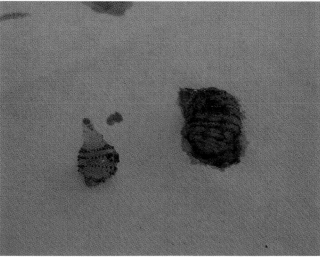

Botfly infestations are notably common in South America, Mexico, and Central America, especially Belize. Irrespective of the race or ethnicity, travelers to such endemic areas may acquire infection with *Dermatobia hominis,* carried by mosquitos that transfer the eggs, which turn into maggots. The surface of the lesion is characterized by a circular opening through which the maggot extrudes its air hole (Fig. 13.35). When the lesion is poked, the maggot will withdraw into the space. Clearance can be accomplished by surgical removal (Figs. 13.36, 13.37) or by smothering lesions.

Chicken Pox (Figs. 13.38 and 13.39)

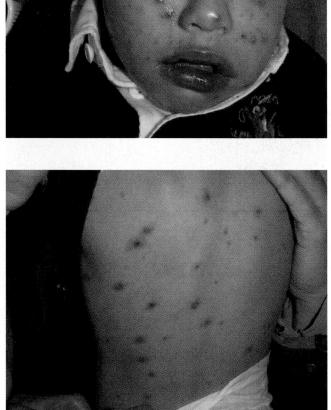

Varicella zoster infection is a highly contagious human herpesvirus infection. While vaccination with a mild strain is effective at preventing wild-type disease, cases are still noted in individuals who were not vaccinated or for whom vaccination immunity waned. Milder and atypical cases are usual for prior vaccines. In the heretofore unvaccinated Asian boy in Figs. 13.38 and 13.39, full blown varicella has erupted affecting the scalp, face, torso, and buttocks. Lesions are itchy to painful vesicles (solitary) on an erythematous base, the so-called dewdrop on a rose petal. Lesions are contagious through contact and aerosolization from 2 days prior to disease appearance until crusting occurs. Accompanying fever, malaise, and upper respiratory symptoms are common.

In Caucasian and Asian children, lesions are prominently erythematous and heal with anetodermic scarring. In children of color, lesions are violaceous and heal with hypertrophic, keloidal, or pitted scarring. Treatment of scarring with resurfacing lasers, microdermabrasion, and fillers has been described [14,15]. The advent of vaccination has minimized cases of varicella pneumonia and encephalitis.

Scarlet Fever (Figs. 13.40, 13.41, 13.42, 13.43)

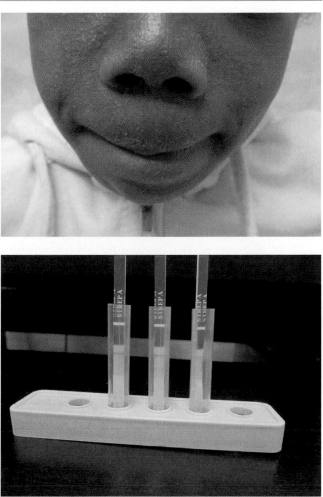

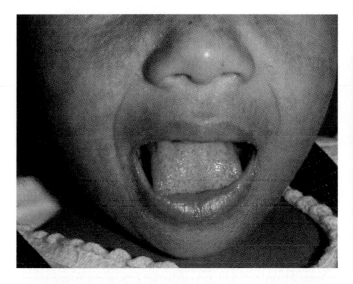

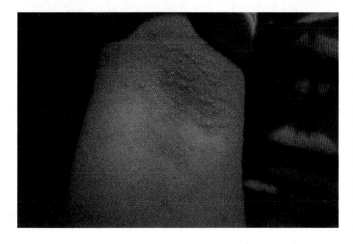

Scarlet fever is a constellation of rash, and fever caused by upper respiratory infection with Group A beta Hemolytic *Streptococcus Pyogenes*. The strep releases toxins that cause the eruption which appears as small papules, which are erythematous in Caucasians and more subtle in darker patients due to the flesh-colored appearance. Similar to the strawberry tongue of Kawasaki's, but lacking in the white coating, the red strawberry tongue of scarlet fever is present in all races and ethnicities (Fig. 13.40). Due to the relative hypopigmentation of the oral mucosa in darker children, the erythema of the tongue is easily noted universally. Prompt antibiotic therapy is needed, even when fever is not present, to avert the sequelae of untreated streptococcal disease.

Clues in all skin tones include the rough or sandpaper feel, the presence of tonsillitis, cervical lymphadenopathy, and a red strawberry tongue. Pastia's lines (Fig. 13.41) are the easiest clinical finding, as they are present in all races and ethnicities. In Pastia's lines, the papules are noted to line up within the skin folds especially in the neck and antecubital region, as shown in this photo. Other sites affected include the axillae and groin. Some children do not mount a fever with scarlet fever. This afebrile variant has the same eruption but diagnosis can be missed. I have yet to see a child in my practice with afebrile scarlet fever who was not Black or Hispanic.

Post-scarlet fever desquamation is often noted after defervescence. When patients mount a low febrile response, confusion in diagnosis is often obviated by this desquamation (Fig. 13.42). Rapid strep test in the second figure shows positive for strep (2 lines) matching the positive control (Fig. 13.43). Institution of therapy is important to prevent post-streptococcal sequelae.

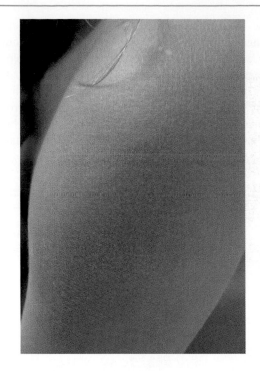

Viral Exanthems Fifth's Disease (Figs. 13.44, 13.45, 13.46)

Fifth's disease is caused by B19 parvovirus, a single stranded DNA virus. Fifth's disease appears with fever followed by an erythematous cheek (slapped cheeks, Fig. 13.44) and a lacy eruption over the proximal extremities (Figs. 13.45 and 13.46). These eruptions are difficult to note in children of color. Black children with sickle cell disease and fetuses of pregnant moms in the second trimester may experience rapid reductions in hematocrits that are life threatening, when exposed to B19 parvovirus. The papular glove and stocking eruption may be caused by B19 parvovirus as well. Due to involvement of the extremities and the relative hypopigmentation of the extremities in children of color, the acral eruption of papular glove and stocking disease is similar in all races, colors, and ethnicities. However, differentiation from infantile acropustulosis is difficult in younger children, with fever and acute onset without itching being fair clues.

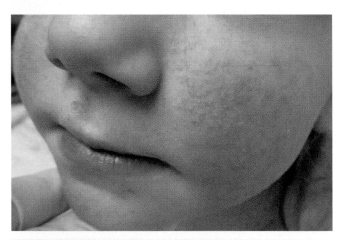

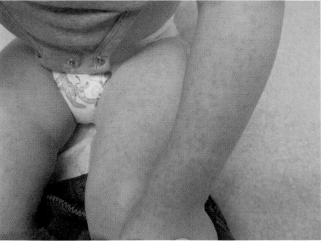

Impetigo (Fig. 13.47)

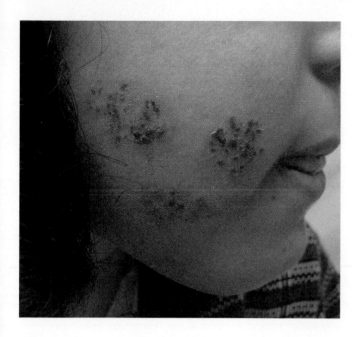

Cutaneous bacterial infections are common in childhood irrespective of race and ethnicity. *Staphylococcus aureus,* more so than *Streptococcus,* causes impetigo. Many children with lesions in the periorificial area carry bacteria in their nasal mucosa. Lesions in Caucasian children demonstrate honey-colored crusts (Fig. 13.47), but the skin tone in darker-skinned children may obscure the color, presenting with purple-brown crusting instead. Similar differences in lesion coloration arise in blistering disorders including herpes virus infections (e.g., Fig. 8.15) and primary blistering diseases.

References

1. Jacyk WK, De Villiers EM (1993) Epidermodysplasia verruciformis in Africans. Int J Dermatol 32:806–810
2. Silverberg NB (2004) Human papillomavirus infections in children. Curr Opin Pediatr 16:402–409
3. Child FJ, Fuller LC, Higgins EM, Du Vivier AW (1999) A study of the spectrum of skin disease occurring in a black population in south-east London. Br J Dermatol 141:512–517
4. Alexis AF, Sergay AB, Taylor SC (2007 Nov) Common dermatologic disorders in skin of color: a comparative practice survey. Cutis 80(5):387–394
5. Martins EL, Gonçalves CA, Mellone FF, Paves L, Tcherniakovsky M, Montes M, Neto M, Pires Sda R, Zequi Sde C, Lacaz CS (1989) Prospective study of pityriasis versicolor incidence in a population of the city of Santo André (state of São Paulo). Med Cutan Ibero Lat Am 17:287–291
6. Frieden IJ, Howard R (1994) Tinea capitis: epidemiology, diagnosis, treatment, and control. J Am Acad Dermatol 31:S42–S46
7. Coley MK, Bhanusali DG, Silverberg JI, Alexis AF, Silverberg NB (2011) Scalp hyperkeratosis and alopecia in children of color. J Drugs Dermatol 10:511–516
8. Williams JV, Eichenfield LF, Burke BL, Barnes-Eley M, Friedlander SF (2005) Prevalence of scalp scaling in prepubertal children. Pediatrics 115:e1–e6
9. Olsen EA, Callender V, McMichael A, Sperling L, Anstrom KJ, Shapiro J, Roberts J, Durden F, Whiting D, Bergfeld W (2011) Central hair loss in African American women: incidence and potential risk factors. J Am Acad Dermatol 64:245–252
10. Kiken DA, Sekaran A, Antaya RJ, Davis A, Imaeda S, Silverberg NB (2006) White piedra in children. J Am Acad Dermatol 55:956–961
11. Jones AL, Koerner RJ, Natarajan S, Perry JD, Goodfellow M (2008) Dietzia papillomatosis sp. nov., a novel actinomycete isolated from the skin of an immunocompetent patient with confluent and reticulated papillomatosis. Int J Syst Evol Microbiol 58:68–72
12. Berk DR (2011) Confluent and reticulated papillomatosis response to 70% alcohol swabbing. Arch Dermatol 147:247–248
13. Silverberg NB, Jackson RM, Laude TA, Tunnessen WW Jr (1998) Picture of the month. Cutaneous larva migrans (creeping eruption). Arch Pediatr Adolesc Med 152:203–204
14. Goel A, Krupashankar DS, Aurangabadkar S, Nischal KC, Omprakash HM, Mysore V (2011) Fractional lasers in dermatology – current status and recommendations. Indian J Dermatol Venereol Leprol 77:369–379
15. Kasper DA, Cohen JL, Saxena A, Morganroth GS (2008) Fillers for postsurgical depressed scars after skin cancer reconstruction. J Drugs Dermatol 7:486–487
16. Pomeranz AJ, Sabnis SS, McGrath GJ, Esterly NB (1999) Asymptomatic dermatophyte carriers in the households of children with tinea capitis. Arch Pediatr Adolesc Med 153:483–486
17. Sharma V, Silverberg NB, Howard R, Tran CT, Laude TA, Frieden IJ (2001) Do hair care practices affect the acquisition of tinea capitis? A case-control study. Arch Pediatr Adolesc Med 155:818–821
18. Chen C, Koch LH, Dice JE, Dempsey KK, Moskowitz AB, Barnes-Eley ML, Hubbard TW, Williams JV (2010) A randomized, double-blind study comparing the efficacy of selenium sulfide shampoo 1% and ciclopirox shampoo 1% as adjunctive treatments for tinea capitis in children. Pediatr Dermatol 27:459–462
19. Greer DL (2000) Successful treatment of tinea capitis with 2% ketoconazole shampoo. Int J Dermatol 39:302–304
20. Silverberg NB (2008) Easy griseofulvin dosing. Pediatr Dermatol 25:577

Acanthosius Nigricans and Stigmata of Metabolic Syndrome (Figs. 14.1–14.3)

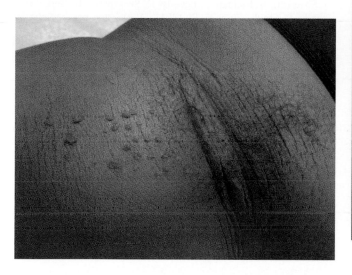

and elbows can be seen with prolonged or advanced cases, but are not as common in adolescents as they are in adults.

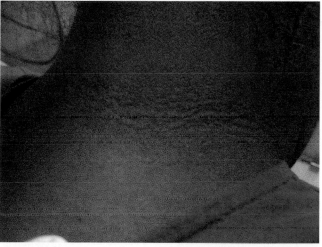

Acanthosis nigricans is a velvety ruggose thickening of the folds of the skin – usually the neck and axillae. In Fig. 14.1, the Hispanic boy with type 2 diabetes mellitus, due to insulin resistance, we note thick acanthosis nigricans with overlying skin tags. Numerous skin tags can be a marker of insulin resistance as well. In a Caucasian child, acanthosis nigricans is tan to light brown velvety rugose thickening of the neck and/or axillary skin, mimicking the light tan lesion of confluent and reticulated papillomatosis of Gougerot and Carteaud (Fig. 13.21), but for location.

The African American girl in Fig. 14.2 with acanthosis nigricans of the neck and insulin resistance has inframammary lesions as well. Eccentric placement of acanthosis nigricans on the face (mid-cheek), inframammary and over the knees

Caucasian teens with acanthosis nigricans have greater body mass index and fasting insulin than Caucasian teens without acanthosis nigricans [1]. A study of children demonstrated that acanthosis nigricans is more common in African American than Caucasian children in the United States, but that independent of race, children with acanthosis nigricans had higher body mass index and fat mass, and that 80% of children with glucose > or = 15 µU/mL had body mass index > or = 3 [2]. Prevalence of acanthosis nigricans in Hispanic/Latino children is also common, but may vary by region. A recent study has suggested that there may be greater risk of metabolic syndrome features among obese children (Table 14.1) from Mexican and Puerto Rican ancestry than in Dominican children [3,4].

Dermatologic Findings or Diseases That Have Been Linked to Obesity [5]

Table 14.1

Acanthosis nigricans
Acne Keloidalis Nuchae (see Fig. 2.29)
Androgenetic alopecia (female pattern in male patient) (Fig. 14.3)
Atopic dermatitis (see Chap. 8) [6]
Cutaneous infections (see Chap. 13) [3]
Granular parakeratosis
Hirsutism
Intertrigo [7]
Keratosis pilaris (See Chap. 8)
Psoriasis vulgaris (see Chap. 6)
Skin tags
Striae distensae (see Chap. 10)

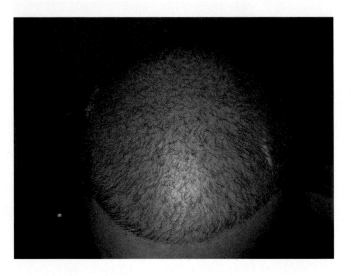

References

1. Aswani R, Lochow A, Dementieva Y, Lund VA, Elitsur Y (2011) Acanthosis nigricans as a clinical marker to detect insulin resistance in caucasian children from West Virginia. Clin Pediatr (Phila) 50(11):1057–1061
2. Nguyen TT, Keil MF, Russell DL, Pathomvanich A, Uwaifo GI, Sebring NG, Reynolds JC, Yanovski JA (2001) Relation of acanthosis nigricans to hyperinsulinemia and insulin sensitivity in overweight African American and white children. J Pediatr 138(4):474–480
3. Stuart CA, Pate CJ, Peters EJ (1989) Prevalence of acanthosis nigricans in an unselected population. Am J Med 87(3):269–272
4. Sherry N, Hassoun A, Oberfield SE, Manibo AM, Chin D, Balachandar S, Pierorazio P, Levine LS, Fennoy I (2005) Clinical and metabolic characteristics of an obese, Dominican, pediatric population. J Pediatr Endocrinol Metab 18(11):1063–1071
5. Shipman AR, Millington GW (2011) Obesity and the skin. Br J Dermatol 165:743–750
6. Silverberg JI, Kleiman E, Lev-Tov H, Silverberg NB, Durkin HG, Joks R, Smith-Norowitz TA (2011) Association between obesity and atopic dermatitis in childhood: a case-control study. J Allergy Clin Immunol 127:1180–1186
7. Mathur AN, Goebel L (2011) Skin findings associated with obesity. Adolesc Med State Art Rev 22:146–156, ix

Pityriasis Lichenoides (Figs. 15.1–15.4)

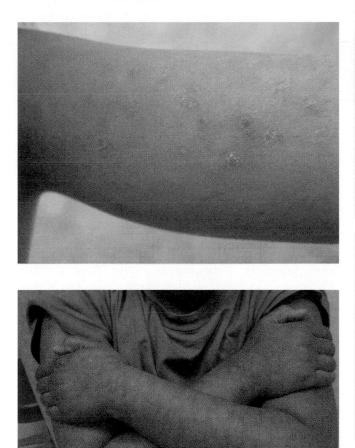

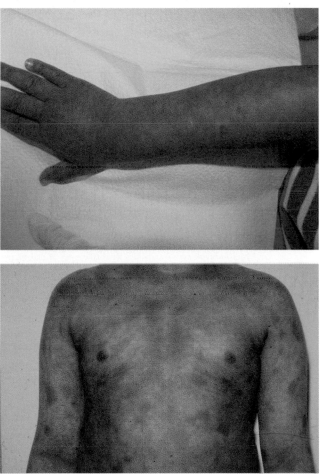

Pityriasis lichenoides is a lymphocytic proliferation in the skin of unknown cause. Two variants exist, pityriasis lichenoides et varioliformis acuta (PLEVA) (also known as Mucha-Habermann disease (MHD)) and chronicum (PLC).

In Asian patients, in PLEVA, there are lymphocytes expressing CD8 and T-cell intracellular antigen-1, whereas CD4+ lymphocytes and FOXP3-positive regulatory T-cells are more abundant in PLC [1]. Clonal T-cell rearrangements are noted in 57% of PLEVA cases and 8% of PLC cases, suggesting that PLEVA cases are a benign-clonal variant of PLC [2]. Precipitation by viral infections, e.g., EBV, HIV, has been reported.

Lesions in PLEVA are erythematous macules and papules usually on the trunk and flexural extremities accompanied by necrotic centers and pseudo-vesicles (Fig. 15.1). Lesions are often necrotic centrally, especially in individuals of color. Fine scale can be noted overlying lesions. A rare febrile form is potentially fatal. Pityriasis lichenoides chronicum is usually more papular in nature with less necrosis. Therapies for pityriasis lichenoides include topical corticosteroids for symptomatic improvement, oral antibiotics as anti-inflammatory agents, methotrexate and narrowband UVB.

In individuals of color, lesions of pityriasis lichenoides chronica can be either erythematous lesions or annular hypopigmented patches to plaques (Figs. 15.2–15.4). Lesions can evolve into mycosis fungoides and repeat biopsies are often needed for monitoring [3]. Presence of lesions over the buttocks is an important clue to the potential presence of mycosis fungoides [4]. Narrowband UVB can be quite helpful in improving hypopigmentation, while flattening lesions [5]. Lesions can resemble vitiligo and atypical or unresponsive cases of widespread hypopigmentation in dark patients should be biopsied to rule out pityriasis lichenoides.

Granulomatous inflammation is far more common in Black patients, especially sarcoidosis. One unusual granulomatous reaction that is uncommon is pseudolymphoma. These are often noted in response to infectious agents such as molluscum, cat scratches or to foreign body reactions. Pseudolymphomas appear mostly in Hispanic and Black children (personal observation), but given their overall rarity, comparison is difficult [6].

Mycosis Fungoides (Figs. 15.5 and 15.6)

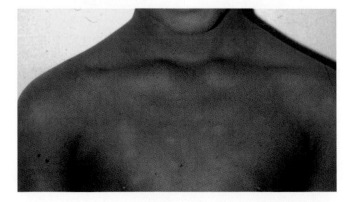

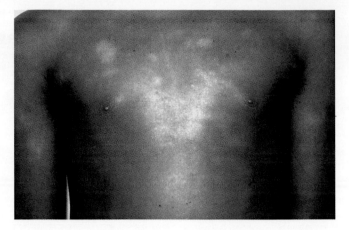

Mycosis fungoides is an indolent form of CD 8+ cutaneous T-cell lymphoma with a good prognosis and normal life expectancy. Onset at age 9 and clinical diagnosis by age 13 years has been reported on average. Most children have patch stage IB cutaneous T-cell lymphoma [7].

In a review of 20 cases of mycosis fungoides in Turkish children, 45% had hypopigmented lesions and 30% purpuric lesions [8]. In Black children, hypopigmentation is even more commonly noted in my experience. In a recent registry of cases from multiple North American and Australian sites, 77% of the children were skin types IV–VI, with 68% having patch stage, 59% manifesting hypopigmentation and 50% with plaque stage [9]. In children of color, lesions are symmetrical hypopigmented, Wood's lamp positive, plaques with subtle atrophy or poikiloderma over the trunk, buttocks and proximal extremities (Figs. 15.5 and 15.6).

Biopsy and re-biopsy are often required to make the diagnosis, especially when lesions evolve from pityriasis lichenoides. T-cell gene re-arrangement studies can be done to document clonality. Screening for elevation, lymph nodes and Sezary cells in the blood is performed bi-annually. Phototherapy to reduce clinical appearance and repigment the skin can be done, but cure is not affected. Hypopigmented mycosis fungoides appears to be a variant mostly noted in Hispanic, Indian, Arabic, or Black children [10, 11]. One should always give consideration of possible HTLV1 infection in cases of individuals from the tropics.

References

1. Kim JE, Yun WJ, Mun SK, Yoon GS, Huh J, Choi JH, Chang S (2011) Pityriasis lichenoides et varioliformis acuta and pityriasis lichenoides chronica: comparison of lesional T-cell subsets and investigation of viral associations. J Cutan Pathol 38:649–656
2. Weinberg JM, Kristal L, Chooback L, Honig PJ, Kramer EM, Lessin SR (2002) The clonal nature of pityriasis lichenoides. Arch Dermatol 138:1063–1067
3. Lane TN, Parker SS (2010) Pityriasis lichenoides chronica in black patients. Cutis 85:125–129

4. Ngo JT, Trotter MJ, Haber RM (2009) Juvenile-onset hypopigmented mycosis fungoides mimicking vitiligo. J Cutan Med Surg 13:230–233

5. Tan E, Lim D, Rademaker M (2010) Narrowband UVB phototherapy in children: a New Zealand experience. Australas J Dermatol 51:268–273

6. Del Boz GJ, Sanz A, Martín T, Samaniego E, Martínez S, Crespo V (2008) Cutaneous pseudolymphoma associated with molluscum contagiosum: a case report. Int J Dermatol 47(5):502–504

7. Nanda A, AlSaleh QA, Al-Ajmi H, Al-Sabah H, Elkashlan M, Al-Shemmari S, Demierre MF (2010) Mycosis fungoides in Arab children and adolescents: a report of 36 patients from Kuwait. Pediatr Dermatol 27:607–613

8. Yazganoglu KD, Topkarci Z, Buyukbabani N, Baykal C (2011) Childhood mycosis fungoides: a report of 20 cases from Turkey. J Eur Acad Dermatol Venereol 2011 Dec 19. doi: 10.1111/j.1468-3083.2011.04383.x. [Epub ahead of print]

9. Pope E, Weitzman S, Ngan B, Walsh S, Morel K, Williams J, Stein S, Garzon M, Knobler E, Lieber C, Turchan K, Wargon O, Tsuchiya A (2010) Mycosis fungoides in the pediatric population: report from an international Childhood Registry of Cutaneous Lymphoma. J Cutan Med Surg 14:1–6

10. Khopkar U, Doshi BR, Dongre AM, Gujral S (2011) A study of clinicopathologic profile of 15 cases of hypopigmented mycosis fungoides . Indian J Dermatol Venereol Leprol 77:167–173

11. Alsaleh QA, Nanda A, Al-Ajmi H, Al-Sabah H, Elkashlan M, Al-Shemmari S, Demierre MF (2010) Clinicoepidemiological features of mycosis fungoides in Kuwait, 1991–2006. Int J Dermatol 49:1393–1398

Index

Printed in the United States of America